SKILLS TRAINING MANUAL FOR DIAGNOSING AND TREATING CHRONIC DEPRESSION

Cognitive Behavioral Analysis System of Psychotherapy

James P. McCullough, Jr.

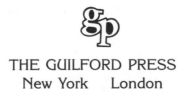

THE GUILFORD PRESS
New York London

Published by The Guilford Press
A Division of Guilford Publications, Inc.
72 Spring Street, New York, NY 10012
www.guilford.com

Printed in the United States of America

The book is printed on acid-free paper.

Last digit is print number: 9 8 7 6 5 4 3 2 1

Library of Congress Cataloging-in-Publication Data

McCullough, James P.
    Skills training manual for diagnosing and treating chronic depression: cognitive behavioral analysis system of psychotherapy / James P. McCullough, Jr.
        p. ; cm.
    Includes bibliographical references.
    ISBN 1-57230-691-2 (pbk.: alk. paper)
    1. Depression, Mental—Diagnosis—Examinations, questions, etc. 2. Depression, Mental—Treatment—Examinations, questions, etc. 3. Cognitive therapy—Handbooks, manuals, etc. I. McCullough, James P. Treatment for chronic depression. II. Title.
    [DNLM: 1. Depressive Disorder—diagnosis—Examination Questions. 2. Depressive Disorder—diagnosis—Handbooks. 3. Cognitive Therapy—Examination Questions.
4. Cognitive Therapy—Handbooks. 5. Depressive Disorder—therapy—Examination Questions. 6. Depressive Disorder—therapy—Handbooks. WM 34 M4787s 2001]
RC537 .M393 2001
616.85′27′0076—dc21   2001033140

In memory of
Henry R. Olivier, MD—
my friend and my first mentor

About the Author

James P. McCullough, Jr., received his PhD from the University of Georgia in 1970. He is a fellow in two divisions (Psychotherapy and Clinical Psychology) of the American Psychological Association. Dr. McCullough was also elected a Diplomate in Clinical Psychology by the American Board of Psychological Forensic Examiners and is director of the Adult Psychotherapy Process Track in the Clinical Training Program at Virginia Commonwealth University (VCU) in Richmond. Currently a Professor of Psychology and Psychiatry and a member of VCU's graduate faculty, he has served since 1972 in the VCU Department of Psychology, where his colleagues gave him the award for Distinguished Research Contribution in Psychology in 2000. Teaching psychotherapy to clinical psychology graduate students has been his overarching educational contribution for the past three decades.

Dr. McCullough's research interests are the chronic depressions—dysthymia, double depression, and chronic major depression. He has conducted research on the diagnostic criteria of the chronic disorders, compared the symptom and psychological characteristics of the chronic disorders to acute/episodic major depression, and gathered empirical treatment/outcome data on more than 250 chronically depressed outpatients. He was a *DSM-IV* Field Trial Coordinator in the American Psychiatric Association's study of dysthymia and major depression. Strongly advocating single-case clinical research that emerges out of practice, Dr. McCullough developed a psychotherapy model, the Cognitive Behavioral Analysis System of Psychotherapy, out of his treatment of chronically depressed outpatients.

Dr. McCullough is the author of many publications, including *Treatment for Chronic Depression: Cognitive Behavioral Analysis System of Psychotherapy*. He founded the Unipolar Mood Disorders Institute at VCU in 1992 and is currently its director.

Preface

The CBASP psychotherapist manual is constructed so that you will learn to administer the therapy model by completing a series of exercises that require therapeutic decisions. In order to make the correct decisions in each exercise, you must first read the parent text, *Treatment for Chronic Depression: Cognitive Behavioral Analysis System of Psychotherapy (CBASP)* (McCullough, 2000). Once you have read the text, you should be ready to tackle the training exercises that will teach you to administer CBASP to chronically depressed patients.

The exercises are designed to teach practitioners how to administer CBASP to criterion level. Answers are provided at the end of each exercise. I hope you will find the exercises challenging and facilitative. I caution against skipping around the manual and working the exercises out of sequence. The learning content in each section presupposes mastery of the earlier sections. Once you have completed the manual, my hope is that you will have learned to react decisively and effectively to the psychopathology of the chronically depressed adult.

It should be noted that the manual is designed specifically for clinicians who treat chronically depressed patients. The manual outline may appear unusual when compared to other therapy manuals available to practitioners. Its difference stems from the exercise format followed throughout. The CBASP manual is designed as a series of exercises so that by the time you have completed all of them, you will know how to make correct decisions about technique administration and patient performance. Why is this so important? I have found that adhering to CBASP methodology in a criterion manner leads to behavior change—nothing is more important than achieving this goal.

Acknowledgments

I am indebted to several people who have provided helpful editorial feedback. Dr. Daniel N. Klein, Professor of Psychology at SUNY at Stony Brook and an individual whom I consider to be the "dean of diagnosticians" when it comes to the chronic disorders, read Chapter Three to check over my course descriptions—I hope these do not disappoint. Drs. Bruce A. Arnow, Associate Professor in the Department of Psychiatry and Behavioral Sciences at Stanford University, and Janice A. Blalock, Assistant Professor at the University of Texas, M. D. Anderson Cancer Center in Houston, reviewed the entire manuscript and worked through each exercise. Their feedback and comments were immensely helpful and led to some necessary changes and clarifications. Two clinical psychologists in the Richmond, Virginia, area—Drs. Teresa A. Buczek and Marilyn N. Spiro—also worked through the exercises and provided me with insightful feedback. Their reactions were beneficial because they approached the manual without formal training in CBASP, and their suggested revisions helped make the manual more user friendly. I am also deeply indebted to my copyeditor, Margaret O. Ryan, for her helpful suggestions and comments, which have resulted in a better overall text. Margaret, who also helped with the editing of the parent text, is a master at word construction, and thanks to her work the end product reads much more smoothly.

Finally, I want to thank Kitty Moore, Executive Editor of The Guilford Press, for her continued encouragement and enthusiastic support.

Contents

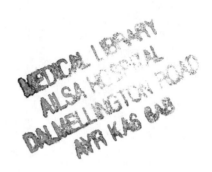

Treating the chronically depressed adult—dislodging the refractory cognitive-emotional and behavioral armor that is the disorder—is analogous to breaking through a granite wall using a 10-pound sledgehammer. One hits the wall repeatedly in the same area, with little or no effect, and then, almost imperceptibly, a slight hairline crack appears. Under continuous pounding, the crack gradually enlarges until, finally, the wall breaks and crumbles.

ONE

Introduction to the Manual

Learning to administer CBASP psychotherapy effectively takes persistence and practice, a thorough understanding of the chronically depressed patient's unique psychopathology, familiarity with the administration of the CBASP techniques, and supervision by a certified trainer. The parent text for this manual, *Treatment for Chronic Depression: Cognitive Behavioral Analysis System of Psychotherapy (CBASP)* (McCullough, 2000), discusses the psychopathology of the patient and thoroughly describes the CBASP techniques. This manual is designed to be a training companion to the book. By working through the exercises in the manual, you will learn how to diagnose the chronically depressed patient and to administer the CBASP techniques.

The *starting point* for CBASP trainees is understanding the pathology of the patient. I cannot state this point strongly enough! The chronic population is *not* similar to patients with acute/episodic major depression. The CBASP techniques will make sense only if you understand the idiosyncratic problems of chronic patients. Beginning psychotherapists must embark on their CBASP training by reading the parent text, *Treatment for Chronic Depression: Cognitive Behavioral Analysis System of Psychotherapy* (McCullough, 2000). Whenever references to this book are inserted in the manual, the book is referred to as "the text." Even experienced therapists should complete the text before beginning this manual.

The manual is divided into five chapters. Chapter One describes the organizational format. Chapter Two presents a brief review of the psychopathology of chronic depression, a general description of the therapy model, and the outcome goals of therapy. Chapter Three teaches a method of graphing the clinical course of chronic patients so that you can discriminate the chronic disorders from those of acute/episodic major depression. Chapters Four and Five describe how to administer the CBASP techniques.

The most important CBASP technique is Situational Analysis (SA), which is designed to move the patient from a preoperational level of cognitive-emotional functioning to a formal level. The Interpersonal Discrimination Exercise (IDE) is weighted second in importance, and Behavioral Skill Training/Rehearsal (BST/R) is ranked third. (BST/R is not covered in the manual but these learning exercises are reviewed and discussed in detail in CBASP Training Workshops. Workshop dates are announced in professional journals and newsletters, at annual national professional conventions, and at state and local psychological and psychiatric association meetings.)

Ranking the techniques is a necessary evil to facilitate structuring the session. Do not, however, take my comments as "gospel" and rigidly structure each therapy hour to adhere to my rankings. Would that the psychotherapy process be so cut and dry. Obviously, a number of exigencies make rigid adherence to any technique rankings unproductive: the ebb and flow of issues from session to session, the fact that an SA conducted during an early session may not be completed in one sitting and may have to be continued at the next meeting, and/or the fact that an interpersonal crisis can arise and require an extended focus for one or more hours. The weightings that I propose reflect the proportion of in-session time per technique that I think will be most productive over the course of the entire therapy process. I recommend that the majority of the hour (e.g., 75%) be spent doing SA, with about 15% of the time devoted to the IDE exercise and 10% to the BST/R. The weighting recommendations are illustrated in Figure 1. You will quickly discover that the actual time you spend administering each technique will vary from week to week. However, strive to give SA the greatest time allocation as much as possible.

If you are feeling overwhelmed by the "size" of the manual—at what looks like an impossible mountain to climb—let me assure you that size is misleading in this case. You will move through the exercises quickly and receive instant feedback for each performance task. I hope the feedback will be both reinforcing and enjoyable. My desired outcome for you is that upon completion, you will be very familiar with the methodology of CBASP. I think you will.

I also wanted to make the exercises rich in clinical relevance as well as sufficiently difficult to be interesting—yet not so hard as to result in frustration and failure. One trainee wrote me this note after completing all of the manual exercises:

> "My experience was that the exercises were fun to do and time went quickly. . . . The exercises were also richly satisfying in their clinical relevance. As I read the SA scenarios, I was reminded time and again of patients of mine who presented situations in similar ways with similar preoperational, self-defeating interpretations of their behavior and life experiences. As a therapist, I found it empowering to work on strategies that could help these patients change."

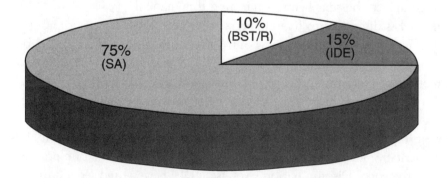

FIGURE 1. Recommended percentage of time spent in psychotherapy session administering three CBASP behavior change techniques.

EXERCISE FORMAT OF THE MANUAL

The diagnostic procedures and CBASP techniques are taught using a series of step-by-step, paper-and-pencil exercises. While readers are learning step-by-step to administer a particular CBASP technique, they can also evaluate and check their work after each exercise is completed. Answers are provided at the end of each training section.

The exercises in Chapter Three focus on making differential diagnoses between chronic depression and acute/episodic major depression. The exercises in Chapters Four and Five deal with modifying the patient's behavior . The exercise format for Chapters Four (SA) and Five (IDE) is shown below:

1. Review the description of the patient's or therapist's performance for a particular step.
2. Write out your answers to the questions that follow.
3. Then check your written work with the answers provided in the manual. If you do not understand my feedback, consult the CBASP text for further information.

Learning will be enhanced if you finish one set of exercises and self-correct any mistakes before moving on to the next set of exercises. *Do not skip around the manual and work randomly. All exercises build on prior learning.*

TWO

"The Big Picture": A Brief Introduction to CBASP

CBASP addresses the severe developmental-structural problems of chronically depressed adults. Preoperational functioning (Piaget, 1926, 1954/1981) is the essential structural characteristic of these patients, and as such, it is the pervasive cognitive-emotional dilemma that affects every area of functioning. Preoperational functioning precludes normal functioning and consigns the individual to (1) chronic failure in coping, (2) intense feelings of helplessness/hopelessness, and (3) a refractory state of depression.

An important aspect of the patient's preoperational dilemma is the fact that he/she is *perceptually disengaged* from his/her environment. Perceptual disengagement from the world one lives in leads to a disordered and rigid behavioral state in which the environment loses its formative power to modify behavior. Chronic patients, unable to change, live out a destructive lifestyle characterized by behavioral rigidity and stereotypy.

As described in detail in Chapter Three of the text, *Treatment for Chronic Depression* (McCullough, 2000), perceptual disengagement stems from a structural cognitive-emotional maturational problem. In the social-interpersonal realm, the patient is inextricably stuck in what Piaget (1926, 1954/1981) identified as the second level of cognitive-emotional development: the "preoperational" stage. At the beginning of psychotherapy, the clinician will be treating an adult who is functioning socially and interpersonally like a 4- to 6-year-old child. I must emphasize two points here about preoperational functioning that I also discussed in the text (pp. 40–50). The first point is that one may function socially and interpersonally like a child yet still score high on a general intelligence test. I do not equate social-interpersonal functioning with general intelligence. I have treated very bright professional people who function preoperationally, just like children, in the social-interpersonal arena. The second point is that early-onset chronically depressed adults typically report more dysfunctional developmental histories than do late-onset patients (Horwitz, 2001). Both types end up functioning socially and interpersonally in a preoperational manner, yet they arrive at this maturation position from different directions and present different clinical courses (see text, pp. 47–50).

CBASP attacks the preoperational dilemma by teaching patients to think and function in formal operational ways (Piaget, 1926, 1954/1981; Inhelder & Piaget, 1958)—a cognitive-emotional perceptual set labeled *perceived functionality* (McCullough, 1984, 2000). Perceived functionality is the generalized awareness that one's behavior has specific consequences. To achieve the goal of helping the patient move from his/her preoperational orientation to a formal operations level of functioning, CBASP relies upon a change principle known as "mismatching demands" (Cowan, 1978; Gordon, 1988; Nannis, 1988). The mismatching principle is described below:

> *If cognitive-emotional didactic exercises are presented at a level that matches current functioning (preoperational), then maturational change will not occur. However, if the adult patient is repeatedly asked to function on a level exceeding his/her current level of functioning (i.e., formal operations), then maturational cognitive-emotional growth will take place.*

Both CBASP techniques are designed to make mismatching demands on patients. When successfully administered, the goals for each technique are (1) to enable patients to make structural- perceptual shifts in functioning and (2) to learn to behave in a more age-appropriate manner. Stated another way, the essential goal for each CBASP technique is to make patients perceptually and behaviorally vulnerable to the consequences of their behavior.

We turn now to Chapter Three, which will teach you how to complete successfully the first step in treatment: correctly diagnosing the chronic patient.

THREE

Diagnosing the Chronically Depressed Adult Using a Clinical Course Timeline

For the first time in the history of the *DSMs*, *DSM-IV* (American Psychiatric Association, 1994, p. 388) graphically illustrates the clinical course of the unipolar mood disorders. Putting graphic course profiles in the unipolar mood disorder section was recommended by the *DSM-IV* Field Trial Committee on Major Depression, Dysthymia, and the Minor Depressions (Keller et al., 1995). The Field Trial Committee felt strongly that accurate diagnosis is contingent upon correctly identifying the course of the unipolar disorder.

CBASP has been developed specifically to treat the chronic depressions. Approximately 75% of the acute/episodic disorders can be treated effectively with medication. This is not the case with the chronic disorders, in which the usual response rate to medication is about 55%. Thus, differentiating these patients from acute/episodic depressives and accurately diagnosing chronic depression often results in more effective treatment. It is for this reason that before you begin the CBASP treatment exercises, you must start with several *DSM-IV* exercises to become sensitized to the importance of the differential diagnostic task.

The text (pp. 51–58) describes the six course patterns of the chronic disorders. In order to determine if the patient has an episodic major depression or meets criteria for one of the six chronic disorders, three diagnostic questions must be answered:

1. Is the present disorder an episodic/acute type of major depression lasting a minimum of two weeks but less than two years?
2. Does the present disorder represent a condition that has lasted for 2 years or more?
3. If the patient is currently diagnosed with a major depressive disorder, is there a history of dysthymia prior to the current episode?

Note: The DSM-IV (American Psychiatric Association, 1994) criteria for dysthymia and major depression will be presented later in this chapter; they are thus positioned so that you can conveniently refer to the *DSM-IV* diagnostic criteria while completing the diagnostic exercises.

The major learning tasks in Chapter Three are (1) determining whether the depressive course is episodic/acute or chronic and (2) whether or not antecedent dysthymia is present. With episodic/acute unipolar cases, clinicians will probably begin treatment using one of the newer SSRIs (selective serotonin reuptake inhibitors). When the presenting problem (usually major depression) is diagnosed as having a chronic course, combination treatment (medication and psychotherapy) should be the treatment of choice (Keller et al., 2000).

If antecedent dysthymia is diagnosed, then a brief reevaluation for the continued presence of dysthymia is necessary once the patient's major depression has remitted. The practitioner must determine if there has been a 2-month period during which the patient has been free of dysthymic symptoms. A lingering dysthymic condition that is either unidentified and/or untreated increases the probability (up to 90%) of a relapse into another major depressive episode within one year (Keller, 1988, 1990; Keller & Hanks, 1994; Keller, Lavori, Rice, Coryell, & Hirschfeld, 1986). The recommended procedure for determining the course of chronic depression and for identifying the presence of antecedent dysthymic disorder follows.

INTRODUCTION TO THE DEPRESSION TIMELINE WORKSHEET

Once the presenting problem is diagnosed as a unipolar depressive disorder (either major depression or dysthymic disorder), the next step is to determine the duration of the current disorder (e.g., "How long have you felt the way you feel *right now?*"). If after the initial diagnosis is made, the clinician sees that the current episode has lasted longer than 6 months, I recommend using the *Depression Timeline Worksheet* (see Figure 2) (McCullough et al., 1996) to identify the clinical course. The worksheet will illustrate the variations in symptom intensity in a patient's depression over the preceding 2 years (and beyond, if necessary).

In constructing the depression timeline, clinicians should work collaboratively with patients. A clipboard is a practical surface to use, as it can be passed back and forth easily between patient and therapist. The following steps are recommended in order to complete the Timeline Worksheet:

1. The collaborative assistance of the patient should be obtained.

   The clinician explains that the purpose of the exercise is to determine the history of the patient's disorder. Continuing to explain, he/she says that the history of the depression is important to know because the diagnosis of the disorder and the subsequent treatment are both determined by the historical information.

2. The Timeline is completed working from left to right across the severity grid. The lettered row above the severity grid represents calendar months from right to left.

   Begin with the year and month the diagnostic interview is conducted (i.e., January = J, February = F, March = M, and so on). If, for example, the screening month is "August 1999," the *starting point* on the grid would be five slots from the left under "A" for August. Enter the year the screening interview is conducted in the space provided.

3. The current diagnosis determines the "severity rating" on the Timeline Worksheet. The severity levels on the grid are rated as follows:

INSTRUCTIONS

1. Work from left to right and mark "X's" under the appropriate months.
2. Start by writing current year; begin rating in current month.
3. Use Timeline I to establish chronic course of present disorder.
4. Use Timelines II and III to plot course over the life span (note "years" as much as possible).

Year of screening interview _____

MONTHS |D|N|O|S|A|J|J|M|A|M|F|J|D|N|O|S|A|J|J|M|A|M|F|J|D|N|O|S|A|J|J|M|A|M|F|J

I.
Normal
Mild
Moderate
Severe

II.
Normal
Mild
Moderate
Severe

III.
Normal
Mild
Moderate
Severe

Diagnosis of patient: _____   Early/Late-onset: _____

FIGURE 2. Depression Timeline Worksheet used to graph clinical course.

Normal: No symptoms of depression present.

Mild: Dysthymic disorder *or* a decrease in the intensity of a major depressive episode below syndromal threshold.

Moderate: Major depression (mild-to-moderate in severity and rated as such by a reported *just noticeable impairment level* in work, family, and/or social functioning).

Severe: Major depression (*significant/obvious impairment* in work, family, and/or social functioning reported).

Examples for a *mild* rating: Patient discloses: "not doing as well as I used to," "not going out as much as I used to," "not as attentive to my wife and family as I used to be—just don't feel like it," etc.

Examples for a *moderate* rating: Patient states that others are noticing a change in behavior due to his/her mood and suggesting either verbally or nonverbally, that something is wrong with him/her: "You don't seem to want to go out anymore—something seems to be bothering you."; "Your work has not been as good lately. Is it because you're feeling bad or depressed?"; "Daddy, you watch TV a lot—you don't do anything with us any more."

Examples for *severe* rating: Patient actually misses work, skips classes, stops dating, or disrupts the usual family routines by active withdrawal, heightened irritability, etc.

4. "Personalize" the Timeline by working from left to right and by beginning at the month the diagnostic interview is conducted.

For example, ask the patient to write in or report significant and personal events in the month slots for the previous 2 years (e.g., anniversaries, birthdays, religious holidays, births, deaths, national holidays, marriage, divorce, etc.) and any other positive or negative family, social, or national events that will enhance the retrospective recall of mood.

5. Place an "X" in the slot indicating the current severity of the disorder beginning with the diagnostic interview month. Note: You will be working back in time, from left to right on the grid. The sequence of months reflects this time orientation and runs from December to January.

The first "X" functions as the *comparative severity anchor-point* that will be used to rate depression severity levels as you move back in time. After the anchor-point is set, ask the patient:

a. "How long have you felt this way, the way you are feeling right now?"

Once the duration and severity of the current episode is established, the next inquiry concerns what happened to the severity level at the change point: Did the severity increase or decrease? Ask the patient:

b. "At this point, were you depressed or did you feel more or less depressed compared to how you feel now?"

Whenever the patient recalls a shift in depression severity, mark an "X" on the grid under the appropriate month. *The same question concerning duration is asked at each change point in severity*. When the exercise is completed, connect the "X's" with a line and the course profile of the chronic disorder will be evident.

Note: Once the severity level for major depression is set at either a *mild*, *moderate*, or *severe* level, decreases in depression intensity over time are always rated on the Timeline at a *mild* level. These periods represent times when a "partial recovery" is experienced. If the patient reports no symptoms for 8 weeks or longer at his/her severity change points, then the rating should be marked *normal* (denoting "full recovery" from the Major Depression).

At this point, we are *not* trying to diagnose a dysthymic disorder unless the *mild* ratings remain in place for 2 years or more and a major depression does not occur within 2 years of the onset of the milder disorder. Most double depression patients (antecedent dysthymia followed by one or more episodes of major depression: Keller & Shapiro, 1982, 1984) report an early onset of dysthymia (mild rating on the grid) at about 15 years of age.

Note: Statements typical of early-onset dysthymic disorder at screening are: "I've always felt down," "Feeling depressed is normal for me," "I've been depressed for as long as I can remember," and so on. Approximately 75% of early-onset dysthymic patients report an insidious onset pattern; that is, they are unable to pinpoint any one precipitating event that caused the depression.

The time limits of the worksheet are for convenience only. Using the current diagnosis as the comparative severity anchor-point, the clinician can easily extend the course exercise over the life span.

6. If it appears that antecedent dysthymia is a precursor to the current episode of major depression because the patient is recalling a 2-year period (or more) of mild depression, try to pinpoint the onset age of the milder disorder.

   One of the most frequent course patterns that occurs among double depression patients is a recurrent pattern of major depressive episodes that returns to the dysthymia baseline (*DSM-IV*: "without full interepisode recovery," p. 388, American Psychiatric Association, 1994) between episodes.

7. Patients diagnosed with dysthymic disorder at screening ("X" = mild severity) should be asked:

   a. "*How long* have you felt the way you are feeling right now?"
   b. "Was there *ever a time* when you felt more depressed than you feel right now, or when your depression deepened in intensity?"
   c. "*When* was this?"
   d. "*How long* did you feel this way?"
   e. "*Before that*, did you feel about the way you are feeling right now?"

If the patient answers "yes" to the first question, and there were periods of 2 weeks or longer when the patient experienced major depressive episodes, the timeline should denote one or more "troughs/dips" reflecting the periods when the major depressive episodes interrupted the course of the dysthymic disorder.

DSM-IV CRITERIA FOR MAJOR DEPRESSION AND DYSTHYMIC DISORDER

Before you practice diagnosing and graphing the course of the major depressive disorders, a brief review of the *DSM-IV*'s diagnostic criteria for major depression and dysthymic disorder is necessary. Consult the criteria freely when working on the clinical course exercises below.

Criteria for dysthymic disorder

1. Feeling down/depressed most of the day, more days than not, for the past 2 years.

2. Presence of two (or more) of the following symptoms most of the day, more days than not, for 2 years:

   a. poor appetite or overeating
   b. insomnia or hypersomnia
   c. low energy or fatigue
   d. low self-esteem
   e. poor concentration/difficulty making decisions
   f. feelings of hopelessness

3. No major depressive episode present during the first 2 years of the disturbance.

Criteria for major depressive disorder

1. Five (or more) of the following symptoms have been present most of the day, nearly every day, during the same 2-week period (either *a* or *b* must be present for the diagnosis):

   a. depressed mood
   b. markedly diminished interest/pleasure in all/almost all activities
   c. significant weight loss/gain of 5% of body weight (not dieting/trying to gain weight) during the past month
   d. insomnia or hypersomnia
   e. psychomotor retardation/agitation
   f. fatigue/loss of energy
   g. feelings of worthlessness or excessive/inappropriate guilt
   h. diminished ability to think or concentrate, or indecisiveness
   i. recurrent thoughts of death, suicidal ideation, specific plan for suicide, or specific attempt

Note: Some trainees have found that making extra copies of the timeline exercise page before beginning the diagnostic exercises is useful. These extra sheets can be used if you want to engage in extra practice.

DEPRESSION TIMELINE WORKSHEET EXERCISES

Before beginning the exercises, review the sample exercise, using Figure 3 as a guide.

Example Case

A 38-year-old female patient was diagnosed with major depression, moderate, at the intake interview conducted on May 4, 1999. The patient was assigned a *moderate* rating because she reported that her husband had started encouraging her to see someone about her sad mood. He felt it was not normal for her to be down so much of the time. She also reported not missing any work nor had she slacked off on helping out around the house.

Since the interview was conducted during May of 1999, we will start by entering the year in the space provided. Working from left to right, we will place an "X" under the month of May (the second M) on the row indicating a *moderate* severity rating for her depression.

THERAPIST: I want you to look at this chart. Let's put in some important monthly events for you. Start with your birthday. What is your birthday month?

PATIENT: September.

THERAPIST: All right, let's write in "birthday" above the slot for October. What about your marriage anniversary month?

PATIENT: I got married in January, 1984.

THERAPIST: I'll insert that above the three slots for January in the top row. Are there any other important dates that would help you personalize this timeline?

PATIENT: My family and I always go to Washington, D.C. to watch the fireworks on July 4th. Hanukkah and my two girls' birthdays are important dates. My older girl was born in February and the younger one in June.

THERAPIST: Now as you [the patient] write in these events, your calendar begins to take on a more personal flavor. I think these dates will help you remember how you were feeling as we look back over time. As you look back now, how long have you been feeling the way you are feeling right now?

PATIENT: Let's see, I have been feeling this way since last December 1998. It was Hanukkah and I found out that my husband was seeing another woman. I never found out how long the affair had gone on. He swears he has not seen her since I found out. One of my friends told me she had seen the two of them check into a motel one evening. I have been feeling bad ever since.

THERAPIST: I'm going to put some "X's" on this line through December 1998. You and I are going to keep going back in time. Let me ask you, is this the first time you felt depressed? I mean, were you feeling down or depressed before you found out about your husband's affair in December?

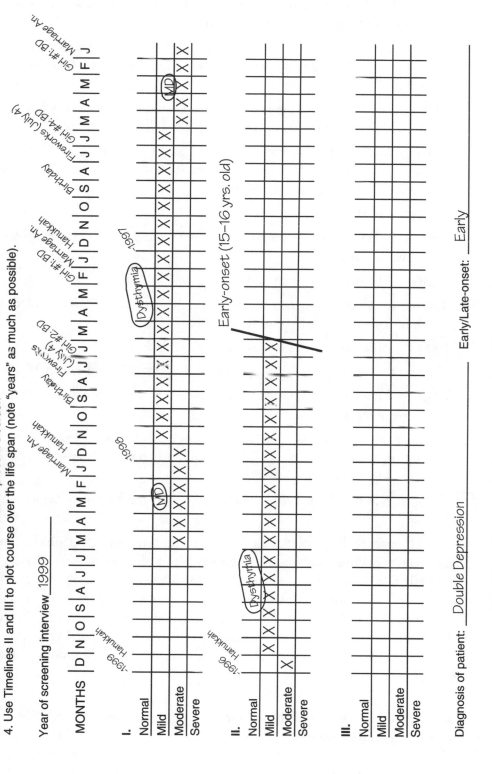

FIGURE 3. Example of a depression Timeline Worksheet for double depression case.

PATIENT: Yes, I have been depressed most of my life. [Remember, this is an expression typical of early-onset dysthymia patients.]

THERAPIST: So this was a worsening of a depression that you had already been feeling. Before you felt more depressed in December 1998, how long had you felt the other way—the less depressed way?

PATIENT: The only other time I felt this bad was during May 1997, when my girlfriend moved out of town, and I was left with no close friends.

THERAPIST: Would it be accurate to mark the graph on the *mild* row. Correct me if I am wrong. If I mark "X's" from November 1998 through June 1997, would this "X-trail" chart the course of your mood?

PATIENT: Yes, that looks accurate.

THERAPIST: When your girlfriend moved in May 1997, was your depression like it is now, or was it worse?

PATIENT: About like it is now.

THERAPIST: Alright, I'll put an "X" in the slot here for May 1997. The next question is, how long did this depression period last?

PATIENT: About 6 months, through December 1996.

THERAPIST: Again, were you depressed before your girlfriend left in May 1997?

PATIENT: I have been depressed since I was about 15 years old. I don't know why. I guess I'm just a weak person.

THERAPIST: I know this is a difficult question, but did your depression ever take a turn for the worse between your 15th year and when your depression became more severe in May 1997?

PATIENT: Not that I can recall. I've just been sad since I can remember.

Final comments: The patient describes a well-known course of double depression with two episodes of major depression. She is currently in a major depressive episode. The early-onset dysthymic disorder began when she was an adolescent. During the periods of remission from the two major depressive episodes, she returned to a dysthymic disorder baseline. We will predict that if the dysthymic disorder and major depression are not both treated to remission, and if the patient does not remain in treatment for several years after full remission of both disorders occur, she will continue to have repeated episodes of major depression throughout her life.

Now that you have reviewed the sample exercise, work through the following exercises and see how you do. These exercises will help you learn how to determine the clinical course of chronic depression. Read the verbatim descriptions carefully and use the timeline grid to chart the patient's course of depression; then write in your diagnosis. (Refer to the diagnostic criteria and severity ratings above as often as you like.)

> **Reminder: The severity levels on the grid are rated as follows:**
>
> *Normal:* No symptoms of depression present.
>
> *Mild:* Dysthymic disorder *or* a decrease in the intensity of a major depressive episode below syndromal threshold.
>
> *Moderate:* Major depression rated by a just noticeable impairment level in work, family, and/or social functioning (e.g., other people are noticing).
>
> *Severe:* Significant/obvious impairment in work, family, and/or social areas (e.g., actually missing work, etc.).

Exercises

Timeline Exercise 1

A 23-year-old patient meets current criteria for major depression, moderate, since he reports not performing "as well as I used to at work, home, and with my friends, and others are beginning to comment on the changes in my behavior." The diagnostic interview was conducted during December of 1998. The patient also said that he had been feeling this depressed for the past 7 months, so the therapist decided to use the Timeline Worksheet.

THERAPIST: How long have you been depressed just like you feel right now?

PATIENT: It's been about 7 months. I lost my job at the factory about June 5th.

THERAPIST: Were you feeling this depressed before you lost the job?

PATIENT: Yes, but not anything like this.

THERAPIST: Prior to June of this year, you say you were feeling depressed but that it was not as bad as you are feeling right now. Can you recall how long you had been feeling this way—the way you were feeling before you lost your job?

PATIENT: Looking back on it now, it was since my sophomore year in high school. I was about 16, and it was during the fall, October or November. Just realized I wasn't happy. Felt that way until last June, when the bottom dropped out on me with this depression.

THERAPIST: Had you ever been aware of feeling down or being unhappy before you were 16?

PATIENT: No.

THERAPIST: Let's look at the period between 16 years old and now. Since you first noticed that you were not feeling happy at about age 16, has your mood ever returned to normal for a period of time when you no longer felt down or depressed?

PATIENT: No.

THERAPIST: Did your depression worsen or deepen before you lost your job in June—say, from the time you were 16 up until this past June?

PATIENT: No.

Directions. Chart the course of this patient's depression on the Timeline on p. 16. Next, diagnose the patient. (*Answers to Exercise 1 can be found on p. 37.*)

INSTRUCTIONS

1. Work from left to right and mark "X's" under the appropriate months.
2. Start by writing current year; begin rating in current month.
3. Use Timeline I to establish chronic course of present disorder.
4. Use Timelines II and III to plot course over the life span (note "years" as much as possible).

Year of screening interview _____

MONTHS |D|N|O|S|A|J|J|M|A|M|F|J|D|N|O|S|A|J|J|M|A|M|F|J

I.

Normal
Mild
Moderate
Severe

II.

Normal
Mild
Moderate
Severe

III.

Normal
Mild
Moderate
Severe

Diagnosis of patient: _____   Early/Late-onset: _____

Timeline Diagnostic Exercise 1

Timeline Exercise 2

The patient is a 38-year-old utility worker who told the therapist, "I have been depressed for as long as I can remember." (With this type of comment, the therapist suspects early-onset dysthymic disorder before the emergence of one or more major depressive episodes.) The patient is diagnosed as currently meeting criteria for major depression, severe. He said he had been missing work 2 to 3 days a week for the past 3 months. The interview was conducted in February 1999.

THERAPIST: How long have you been feeling just the way you are feeling right now?

PATIENT: Since about June of 1998 when my girlfriend and I broke up—let's see, it's been about 9 months.

THERAPIST: Try to remember, were you depressed or feeling down before you broke up with your girlfriend in June of last year? Were you depressed and was it as intense as it is now?

PATIENT: No, I was down, but it was much less intense.

THERAPIST: All right, let's see if we can determine how long this period lasted. How long had you been feeling the way you felt before the breakup last June?

PATIENT: I've felt that way since college—since May 1982. It was my senior year at State when I really got down like I am now. I broke up with another woman at Christmas in, let's see, it was December 1981. I stayed really depressed for a good 6 months, until I graduated and went into the army. I almost didn't graduate because I missed so many classes. I came out of that bad depression stuff in June 1982. I don't know why, I just starting feeling better.

THERAPIST: Again, was your more severe depression in 1981–82 about like you feel right now?

PATIENT: About the same as now.

THERAPIST: Did you feel down or depressed before December 1981?

PATIENT: Yes, I told you, I've been feeling down since I can remember, though not as bad as I feel right now. It must have started in middle school (about 13 years old) when I first noticed I was feeling down. Don't have any idea why I started feeling bad.

Directions. Chart the course of the patient's depression on the Timeline on p. 18. Next, diagnose the patient. (*Answers to Exercise 2 can be found on p. 38.*)

INSTRUCTIONS

1. Work from left to right and mark "X's" under the appropriate months.
2. Start by writing current year; begin rating in current month.
3. Use Timeline I to establish chronic course of present disorder.
4. Use Timelines II and III to plot course over the life span (note "years" as much as possible).

Year of screening interview _____

MONTHS | D | N | O | S | A | J | J | M | A | M | F | J | D | N | O | S | A | J | J | M | A | M | F | J

I.

Normal
Mild
Moderate
Severe

II.

Normal
Mild
Moderate
Severe

III.

Normal
Mild
Moderate
Severe

Diagnosis of patient: _____   Early/Late-onset: _____

Timeline Diagnostic Exercise 2

Timeline Exercise 3

An Asian American male said he became depressed at about 24 years of age when he took his first job in an engineering firm. He is 42 years old now. Upon further questioning, the therapist felt that the patient currently met criteria for major depression, moderate. The patient said he was not missing work, still went out with friends, and continued to be an important part of the family. However, others have noticed changes in his mood and have commented to him about it. He just couldn't shake the depression. The diagnostic interview was held in April 1997.

THERAPIST: How long have you felt the way you are feeling right now?

PATIENT: Gosh, I've felt this way since I was 24 years old. I got married that year (1979), and shortly after the ceremony, I started getting depressed. Right after I married, I realized I was not prepared to live with a woman. I had not dated very much. In fact, Carol, my wife, was the first woman I dated more than one or two times. We had only dated for a month when I asked her to marry me. Well, we got married and then I realized what a mistake I made. I wasn't even sure that I loved her, much less wanted to live with her. Been depressed ever since.

THERAPIST: You say you were 24 years old, got married, and then became depressed. And looking back, you feel that you have been depressed like you are right now since that time?

PATIENT: Nothing much has changed since I was 24.

THERAPIST: Let me ask it another way. Has your depression intensity changed at all since you were 24 years old? That is, have you gone through periods when you were less depressed or when your depression went away for a period of time?

PATIENT: No. It's pretty much been the same since I married.

THERAPIST: Before you got married, did you ever have periods when you felt down or were depressed?

PATIENT: No.

Directions. Chart the course of this patient's depression on the Timeline on p. 20. Next, diagnose the patient. (*Answers to Exercise 3 can be found on p. 39.*)

INSTRUCTIONS

1. Work from left to right and mark "X's" under the appropriate months.
2. Start by writing current year; begin rating in current month.
3. Use Timeline I to establish chronic course of present disorder.
4. Use Timelines II and III to plot course over the life span (note "years" as much as possible).

Year of screening interview _____

MONTHS | D | N | O | S | A | J | J | M | A | M | F | J | D | N | O | S | A | J | J | M | A | M | F | J | D | N | O | S | A | J | J | M | A | M | F | J

I.

Normal
Mild
Moderate
Severe

II.

Normal
Mild
Moderate
Severe

III.

Normal
Mild
Moderate
Severe

Diagnosis of patient: _____   Early/Late-onset: _____

Timeline Diagnostic Exercise 3

> **Reminder: The severity levels on the grid are rated as follows:**
>
> *Normal:*   No symptoms of depression present.
>
> *Mild:*   Dysthymic disorder *or* a decrease in the intensity of a major depressive episode below syndromal threshold.
>
> *Moderate:* Major depression rated by a just noticeable impairment level in work, family, and/or social functioning (e.g., other people are noticing).
>
> *Severe:*   Significant/obvious impairment in work, family, and/or social areas (e.g., actually missing work, etc.).

Timeline Exercise 4

The patient is a 45-year-old married female. She is diagnosed at screening (November 1999) with a major depression, mild. She was discharged from the hospital a month ago (late October) because her depression symptoms were less severe. At hospital admission, she was diagnosed major depression, severe. In early October 1999, she had been admitted to the hospital because of threatening suicidal impulses. The clinician was concerned that suicide was a serious possibility.

THERAPIST: When did you first begin feeling down, the way you were down when you were admitted to the hospital in early October?

PATIENT: It was during the early fall—let's see, around September, when my daughter got married.

THERAPIST: Before September did you feel depressed or down?

PATIENT: Yes, but nothing like I felt when my daughter got married.

THERAPIST: Let's see if we can determine the history of your depression. You mentioned that you felt down before September, but not as bad as you felt after the wedding. How long had you been feeling the way you did before the wedding?

PATIENT: I have felt this way since February of this year. Before that, it was in August 1998, when I had to be hospitalized again for two weeks. My husband got a promotion, and it meant he would be out of town for a week out of every month. I didn't feel I could live without him.

THERAPIST: Let's see if I got it. Between February and September of 1999, you felt less depressed than you felt when you entered the hospital in October of this year. But you felt much more depressed during January. You stated that your depression got much worse in August 1998. Between August 1998 and January 1999, how depressed were you?

PATIENT: I missed a lot of work, and I don't think I was a very good wife or mother.

THERAPIST: Were there times during the August to January period when you were not depressed?

PATIENT: No, I was depressed all the time.

THERAPIST: Can you recall how you felt before August 1998? Did you feel down or depressed before that time?

PATIENT: Yes, I was down, but not as bad.

THERAPIST: Let me ask you the same kind of question as I did before. How long did you feel down this time, say, starting with August 1998 and looking back?

PATIENT: For several years. I was hospitalized when I was 30 because of some problems at work. I just never got over the depression after I was discharged. I think I was hospitalized during the summer of 1984.

THERAPIST: Are you saying that you have been depressed from 1984 to 1998, though not as bad as you felt when you were hospitalized during the summer of 1984?

PATIENT: Yes.

THERAPIST: When was the first time that you noticed being down, feeling sad?

PATIENT: When I was about 24 years old. I broke up with a guy in September 1978. I was supposed to marry him that year. I didn't get up out of bed for two weeks except to eat. For some reason, the depression got better the next month (in October), but it never really went away. Then, it got really bad again in 1984.

Directions. Chart the course of the patient's depression on the Timeline on the facing page. Next, diagnose the patient. (*Answers to Exercise 4 can be found on p. 40.*)

INSTRUCTIONS

1. Work from left to right and mark "X's" under the appropriate months.
2. Start by writing current year; begin rating in current month.
3. Use Timeline I to establish chronic course of present disorder.
4. Use Timelines II and III to plot course over the life span (note "years" as much as possible).

Year of screening interview _____

MONTHS | D | N | O | S | A | J | J | M | A | M | F | J | D | N | O | S | A | J | J | M | A | M | F | J

I.

Normal
Mild
Moderate
Severe

II.

Normal
Mild
Moderate
Severe

III.

Normal
Mild
Moderate
Severe

Diagnosis of patient: _____   Early/Late-onset: _____

Timeline Diagnostic Exercise 4

Timeline Exercise 5

A 29-year-old female chemist was diagnosed with dysthymic disorder in July 1998. At the initial interview she said, "I have been most of my life." The therapist wanted to assess for the occurrence of a major depressive episode(s) during the clinical course of her dysthymia.

THERAPIST: Let me ask you some questions about your depression. How long have you felt just the way you are feeling right now?

PATIENT: The last time I felt worse was during the summer of 1997. I was about 27 at the time and my closest girlfriend and I had a serious argument. We didn't speak to each other for 6 months.

THERAPIST: Can you remember when during the summer of 1997 the argument occurred, and can you describe how depressed you became at that time?

PATIENT: I remember it well. It was on my birthday in June 1997, and I became very depressed. I stopped going out socially for about 3 months: I just hung out in my apartment. I also lost some weight—about 10 pounds—lost my appetite. My other friends became real worried about me and told me I ought to go see my doctor. I did, and she put me on some medication. Actually, the medication helped my depression, and I started feeling better in late September. Didn't get over all my depression, but the worst part of it let up.

THERAPIST: Before June 1997, were you depressed about like you are right now?

PATIENT: I have been depressed like I am right now since I was 19 years old. I was a sophomore in college. The depression just came on me. I don't know why I started feeling this way.

THERAPIST: During the period between your sophomore year and June 1997, did your depression ever deepen like it did following the argument with your girlfriend?

PATIENT: No, it stayed pretty much the same.

THERAPIST: Do you remember ever being depressed before you were a sophomore in college?

PATIENT: No, I don't.

Directions. Chart the course of this patient's depression on the Timeline on the facing page. Next, diagnose the patient. (*Answers for Exercise 5 can be found on p. 41.*)

INSTRUCTIONS

1. Work from left to right and mark "X's" under the appropriate months.
2. Start by writing current year; begin rating in current month.
3. Use Timeline I to establish chronic course of present disorder.
4. Use Timelines II and III to plot course over the life span (note "years" as much as possible).

Year of screening interview _____

MONTHS | D | N | O | S | A | J | J | M | A | M | F | J | D | N | O | S | A | J | J | M | A | M | F | J | D | N | O | S | A | J | J | M | A | M | F | J

I.

Normal
Mild
Moderate
Severe

II.

Normal
Mild
Moderate
Severe

III.

Normal
Mild
Moderate
Severe

Diagnosis of patient: _____   Early/Late-onset: _____

Timeline Diagnostic Exercise 5

Timeline Exercise 6

The patient is a 52-year-old construction worker who was diagnosed with dysthymic disorder at screening in February 1997.

THERAPIST: I want to ask you some questions about your depression. How long have you felt the way you are feeling right now?

PATIENT: I have felt this way all my life. My feeling down goes back about as far as I do. Things were really bad in my family. My father and mother were both alcoholics, and they used to beat my brother and me several times a week. When they were drunk, the beatings were worse. I used to think that I had been born into an insane asylum. I never brought my friends around my house because I was afraid of what my parents might be doing. Daddy would even bring other women to the house while my mother was home. It was god awful. My brother was older and he got the worst of it. He even took beatings that I should have gotten. Once when he was a senior in high school he told Daddy that he couldn't bring a woman in the house. My daddy took a swing at him. My brother ducked and hit Daddy square in the jaw. They never spoke after that. My brother left school and joined the army.

THERAPIST: Did the intensity of your depression ever deepen or worsen for 2 weeks or more?

PATIENT: As I said, I've felt this way since as far back as I can remember. Started when I was in early elementary school. Most of my friends called me "sadsack." They knew something was wrong with me. I guess there really was. Sometimes at night when I was alone I'd wish I had a good family where people loved each other. I'm not sure anyone in my family loved anyone else.

THERAPIST: I have one more question I want to ask you. Has there ever been a period of time when you were not depressed? When you felt okay, without any depression?

PATIENT: No. I sure wish I could say "yes" to that question. . . . I was born to be a loser. Things have been bad for me since I was born. Guess I look sad to you, don't I?

Directions. Chart the course of this patient's depression on the Timeline on the facing page. Next, diagnose the patient. (*Answers to Exercise 6 can be found on p. 42.*)

INSTRUCTIONS

1. Work from left to right and mark "X's" under the appropriate months.
2. Start by writing current year; begin rating in current month.
3. Use Timeline I to establish chronic course of present disorder.
4. Use Timelines II and III to plot course over the life span (note "years" as much as possible).

Year of screening interview _____

MONTHS | D | N | O | S | A | J | J | M | A | M | F | J | D | N | O | S | A | J | J | M | A | M | F | J | D | N | O | S | A | J | J | M | A | M | F | J

I.

Normal
Mild
Moderate
Severe

II.

Normal
Mild
Moderate
Severe

III.

Normal
Mild
Moderate
Severe

Diagnosis of patient: _____   Early/Late-onset: _____

Timeline Diagnostic Exercise 6

27

Reminder: The severity levels on the grid are rated as follows:

Normal: No symptoms of depression present.

Mild: Dysthymic disorder *or* a decrease in the intensity of a major depressive episode below syndromal threshold.

Moderate: Major depression rated by a just noticeable impairment level in work, family, and/or social functioning (e.g., other people are noticing).

Severe: Significant/obvious impairment in work, family, and/or social areas (e.g., actually missing work, etc.).

Timeline Exercise 7

The patient is a 49-year-old male, divorced for 5 years, owner of a florist shop. He was seen for a diagnostic interview in mid-December 1999. He was diagnosed with major depression, moderate, because he had missed no work in the recent past, still went out with friends, and continued to date several women. He also stated during the interview that several of his friends and one woman he was dating had remarked that they were worried about him because he had not been himself lately (had seemed down and less outgoing).

THERAPIST: I will ask you several questions about your depression. Will you tell me how long you have felt the way you feel right now?

PATIENT: I have felt this way since the middle of the year, in 1997—during July of that year, I think.

THERAPIST: You are saying that your depression has pretty much remained the same since that time?

PATIENT: Yes.

THERAPIST: Do you know why you became depressed?

PATIENT: I was about to lose my floral shop because business was so bad. I consulted a lawyer about filing for bankruptcy. I've owned this business for 25 years. It's all I have ever done, all I know. I don't know what I would do if I lost this shop. Anyway, I got depressed at that time.

THERAPIST: And in July 1997 you became depressed and have been feeling this way ever since?

PATIENT: Yes. My physician gave me some depression pills, but I stopped taking them after a few weeks. They never did me any good.

THERAPIST: Before July 1997 were you ever bothered by depression or did you have periods when you felt down?

PATIENT: Never. I've always been a pretty happy guy. Things have really gone sour for me.

Directions. Chart the course of this patient's depression on the Timeline on the facing page. Next, diagnose the patient. (*Answers to Exercise 7 can be found on p. 43.*)

INSTRUCTIONS

1. Work from left to right and mark "X's" under the appropriate months.
2. Start by writing current year; begin rating in current month.
3. Use Timeline I to establish chronic course of present disorder.
4. Use Timelines II and III to plot course over the life span (note "years" as much as possible).

Year of screening interview _____

MONTHS | D | N | O | S | A | J | J | M | A | M | F | J | D | N | O | S | A | J | J | M | A | M | F | J

I.

Normal
Mild
Moderate
Severe

II.

Normal
Mild
Moderate
Severe

III.

Normal
Mild
Moderate
Severe

Diagnosis of patient: _____ Early/Late-onset: _____

Timeline Diagnostic Exercise 7

29

Timeline Exercise 8

The patient is a 51-year-old male who was diagnosed with major depression, moderate, at his screening interview in May 1999. The patient was still functioning in the work, family, and social arenas, though he readily admitted that his performance level in these domains was not as good as it used to be. His supervisor had asked him last week if he was feeling all right. The comment was, "You don't look right—are you feeling okay?"

THERAPIST: How long have you felt the way you are feeling right now?

PATIENT: I've been feeling this way since mid-April of this year.

THERAPIST: Before you became as depressed as you are right now, would you describe yourself as being depressed?

PATIENT: Yes, but not as bad as I am now.

THERAPIST: All right, let's work back from mid-April. How long did you feel the way you felt in mid-April?

PATIENT: About 2 years, say back in March 1997. I had been feeling really depressed. In fact, I missed a great deal of work and sat around the house most of the time doing nothing.

THERAPIST: Starting back in March 1997, how long had you been feeling the deep depression?

PATIENT: It lasted about a month. My son was convicted of drunken driving and had to spend a week in jail. No one in my family has ever gotten even a traffic ticket before. It devastated me.

THERAPIST: So you became really depressed around March 1, 1997?

PATIENT: Yes.

THERAPIST: Can you remember if you were feeling depressed prior to March 1st?

PATIENT: Oh, yes! Just not as bad as the March stuff. I have been feeling bad since I was a young boy. I began feeling down in high school and couldn't shake it.

THERAPIST: I want to ask you a question about the period between March 1, 1997, and when you began to feel down in high school. Did your feeling down ever worsen and did you feel like you did in March 1997, or the way you are feeling now?

PATIENT: No. I just felt down. It never really got bad until 1997, and now since mid-April of this year.

Directions. Chart the course of this patient's depression on the Timeline on the facing page. Next, diagnose the patient. (*Answers to Exercise 8 can be found on p. 44.*)

INSTRUCTIONS

1. Work from left to right and mark "X's" under the appropriate months.
2. Start by writing current year; begin rating in current month.
3. Use Timeline I to establish chronic course of present disorder.
4. Use Timelines II and III to plot course over the life span (note "years" as much as possible).

Year of screening interview _____

MONTHS | D | N | O | S | A | J | J | M | A | M | F | J | D | N | O | S | A | J | J | M | A | M | F | J

I.

Normal
Mild
Moderate
Severe

II.

Normal
Mild
Moderate
Severe

III.

Normal
Mild
Moderate
Severe

Diagnosis of patient: _____   Early/Late-onset: _____

Timeline Diagnostic Exercise 8

Timeline Exercise 9

The patient is a 37-year-old male who was screened in January 2000. He was diagnosed with major depression, moderate. According to his supervisor, who had called him into her office and reviewed his yearly evaluation, his work performance had decreased during the previous 6 months . She wanted him to seek help for his depression because it was affecting his job. It was apparent that his depression had been going on for longer than 6 months, so the clinician constructed a course timeline on him.

THERAPIST: How long have you been feeling just like you are feeling today, right now?

PATIENT: It's been over 3 years. My wife died in October, 1996, and I've never gotten over it. We had been married for 12 years. She was everything I ever wanted. I thought we'd grow old together and be able to look back on a long satisfying life. Frankly, I don't know what to do with myself. I've sorta been lost. I don't want to start dating, though my friends keep telling me I need to. I've stopped seeing my friends. I don't like them nagging me.

THERAPIST: You've been grieving for your wife for almost 39 months.

PATIENT: I've thought about going out, but all I do when I go out is think about her, so I'll ruin the evening for anyone I go out with. Dating is just not worth it for me.

THERAPIST: Did you have any problems with depression before your wife died in October 1996?

PATIENT: I've always been depressed. Been depressed for as long as I can remember. In the army, my buddies called me "sadsack."

THERAPIST: Looking back on your history with depression, did you ever have a period or periods when your depression deepened like it did in October 1996?

PATIENT: No, this is the worst it's ever been.

THERAPIST: When did you first notice that you were feeling sad or down?

PATIENT: It was sometime in high school. I don't remember exactly.

Directions. Chart the course of this patient's depression on the Timeline on the facing page. Next, diagnose the patient. (*Answers to Exercise 9 can be found on p. 45.*)

INSTRUCTIONS

1. Work from left to right and mark "X's" under the appropriate months.
2. Start by writing current year; begin rating in current month.
3. Use Timeline I to establish chronic course of present disorder.
4. Use Timelines II and III to plot course over the life span (note "years" as much as possible).

Year of screening interview _____

MONTHS | D | N | O | S | A | J | J | M | A | M | F | J | D | N | O | S | A | J | J | M | A | M | F | J | D | N | O | S | A | J | J | M | A | M | F | J

I.

Normal

Mild

Moderate

Severe

II.

Normal

Mild

Moderate

Severe

III.

Normal

Mild

Moderate

Severe

Diagnosis of patient: _____   Early/Late-onset: _____

Timeline Diagnostic Exercise 9

33

Timeline Exercise 10

The patient is a 31-year-old female inpatient. She was diagnosed by a clinical staff member in May 1999: major depression, severe. The clinician knew that the patient had been admitted to the hospital twice before, so she administered the Timeline so that an accurate diagnosis could be made.

THERAPIST: How long have you been in the hospital?

PATIENT: I've been here 3 weeks now. Came in the first of May.

THERAPIST: Looking at your depression right now, when did you begin to feel this way?

PATIENT: I had a huge fight with my mother over this guy I've been dating. She called me a "slut," a "whore," and said, "You are nothing but white trash." She thinks the man I'm going with is really a bum and that I've lowered my morals to go out with him.

THERAPIST: When did the argument take place?

PATIENT: The middle of April. I became really depressed right after that, and I was admitted to the hospital on May 1. I wanted to kill myself.

THERAPIST: Thinking back now, were you depressed before you had the fight with your mother?

PATIENT: I'm always feeling a little down, but nothing like this. My psychiatrist says that I always have a few depressive symptoms. I've been on antidepressants since I was 23.

THERAPIST: I see you were hospitalized in February 1998. Did you feel like you do now, or was it different?

PATIENT: Just like I feel now. I felt better when I left the hospital in late February. Felt like my usual self.

THERAPIST: Do you know why you became depressed?

PATIENT: My father was drunk one night and slapped me around. It was over another guy I was dating at the time. He didn't like him, and he ordered me to stop seeing him. I got depressed shortly after the argument. Went to see my doctor the next day, and he put me in the hospital right then.

THERAPIST: Thinking back to February 1998, can you remember if you were down or depressed before the argument with your father?

PATIENT: It was sorta like it was between my hospitalizations. I felt a little bit down, but it was not as bad. I always feel a little bit down. I have since the first time I was hospitalized when I was 23. Let's see, it was 1991.

THERAPIST: What happened to you at that time?

PATIENT: My parents and I had a horrible argument right before I went into the hospital. I wanted to stay in an apartment in town, and they demanded that I live at home. They told me the only reason I wanted to have my own apartment was so I could sleep with guys. They are so unreasonable.

THERAPIST: Had you ever had any problems with depression before your first hospitalization when you were 23?

PATIENT: No, this was the first time I even knew what depression was. This is when I started seeing my psychiatrist for medication. I have been seeing him for medicine ever since. I always seem to feel better when I get out of the hospital—I did that time, too.

THERAPIST: Let's see if I'm hearing you correctly. You first got depressed in 1991 when you were 23. After you were discharged, you felt better and not as depressed, but you still had a few symptoms. Then you became really depressed again in February 1998. Once again, you felt better after you were discharged, but you continued to feel a little down. In April 1999 you had another blowup with your mother, and you started feeling really down. And here you and I are today. Is this summary of your depression history correct?

PATIENT: Yes.

Directions. Chart the course of this patient's depression on the Timeline on p. 36. Next, diagnose the patient. (*Answers to Exercise 10 can be found on p. 46.*)

INSTRUCTIONS
1. Work from left to right and mark "X's" under the appropriate months.
2. Start by writing current year; begin rating in current month.
3. Use Timeline I to establish chronic course of present disorder.
4. Use Timelines II and III to plot course over the life span (note "years" as much as possible).

Year of screening interview _____

MONTHS | D | N | O | S | A | J | J | M | A | M | F | J | D | N | O | S | A | J | J | M | A | M | F | J | D | N | O | S | A | J | J | M | A | M | F | J

I.

Normal

Mild

Moderate

Severe

II.

Normal

Mild

Moderate

Severe

III.

Normal

Mild

Moderate

Severe

Diagnosis of patient: _____   Early/Late-onset: _____

Timeline Diagnostic Exercise 10

INSTRUCTIONS

1. Work from left to right and mark "X's" under the appropriate months.
2. Start by writing current year; begin rating in current month.
3. Use Timeline I to establish chronic course of present disorder.
4. Use Timelines II and III to plot course over the life span (note "years" as much as possible).

Year of screening interview __1998__

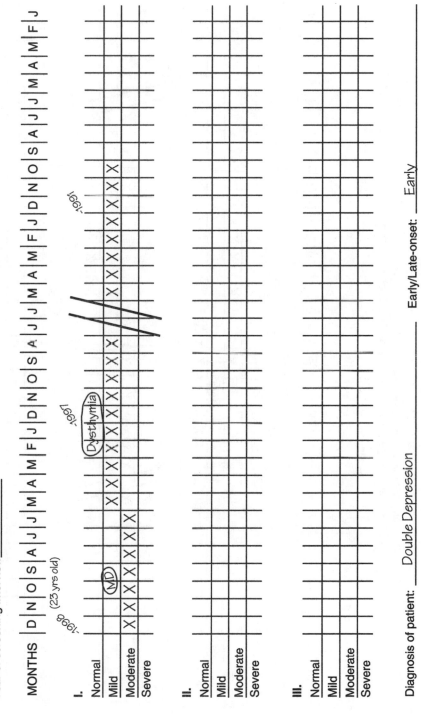

MONTHS | D | N | O | S | A | J | J | M | A | M | F | J | D | N | O | S | A | J | J | M | A | M | F | J | D | N | O | S | A | J | J | M | A | M | F | J

I.

Normal / Mild / Moderate / Severe

(25 yrs old)
-1998
MD
-1997
Dysthymia
-1991

II.

Normal / Mild / Moderate / Severe

III.

Normal / Mild / Moderate / Severe

Diagnosis of patient: __Double Depression__   Early/Late-onset: __Early__

Answers to Diagnostic Exercise 1

INSTRUCTIONS

1. Work from left to right and mark "X's" under the appropriate months.
2. Start by writing current year; begin rating in current month.
3. Use Timeline I to establish chronic course of present disorder.
4. Use Timelines II and III to plot course over the life span (note "years" as much as possible).

Year of screening interview 1999

MONTHS | D | N | O | S | A | J | J | M | A | M | F | J | D | N | O | S | A | J | J | M | A | M | F | J | D | N | O | S | A | J | J | M | A | M | F | J

I.
— 1999 (38 yrs old)
— 1998
— 1997

				Dysthymia
Normal				
Mild		X X X X X X X X X X X X X X X X X X X X X	
Moderate		MD	
Severe	X X X X X X X X		

II.
— 1983
— 1981   Early-onset (13 yrs old)

Normal			
Mild	X X X X X X X X	X X X X X	
Moderate	MD		
Severe	X X X X X X X X X	X X X X X X	

III.

Normal			
Mild			
Moderate			
Severe			

Diagnosis of patient: _____ Double Depression _____   Early/Late-onset: _____ Early

Answers to Diagnostic Exercise 2

38

1. Work from left to right and mark "X's" under the appropriate months.
2. Start by writing current year; begin rating in current month.
3. Use Timeline I to establish chronic course of present disorder.
4. Use Timelines II and III to plot course over the life span (note "years" as much as possible).

Year of screening interview ___1997___

MONTHS |D|N|O|S|A|J|J|M|A|M|F|J|D|N|O|S|A|J|J|M|A|M|F|J|D|N|O|S|A|J|J|M|A|M|F|J

I.

1997
(42 yrs old)

1996

1979

Normal

Mild

Moderate (MD) X X X X X X X X X X (MD) X X X X X X X X X X ?

Severe

II.

Normal

Mild

Moderate

Severe

III.

Normal

Mild

Moderate

Severe

Diagnosis of patient: _____Chronic Major Depression_____ Early/Late-onset: _____Late_____

Answers to Diagnostic Exercise 3

39

INSTRUCTIONS

1. Work from left to right and mark "X's" under the appropriate months.
2. Start by writing current year; begin rating in current month.
3. Use Timeline I to establish chronic course of present disorder.
4. Use Timelines II and III to plot course over the life span (note "years" as much as possible).

Year of screening interview 1999

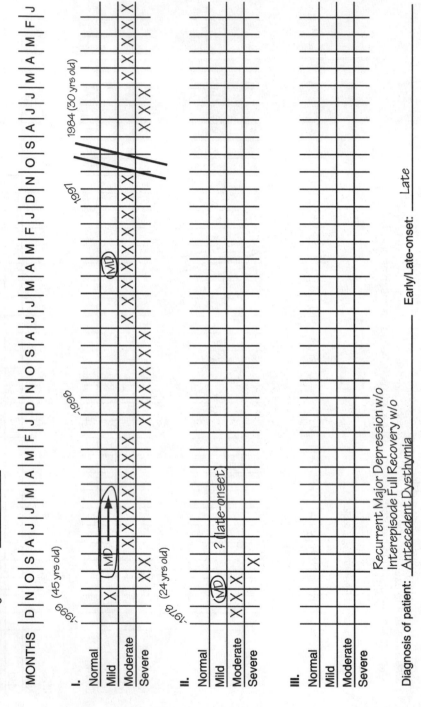

MONTHS | D | N | O | S | A | J | J | M | A | M | F | J | D | N | O | S | A | J | J | M | A | M | F | J

I.
Normal
Mild
Moderate
Severe

—1999 (45 yrs old)
(MD)
—1978 (24 yrs old)
1998
1991
1984 (30 yrs old)

II.
Normal
Mild   ? (late-onset)
Moderate
Severe
(MD)

III.
Normal
Mild
Moderate
Severe

Diagnosis of patient: _Antecedent Dysthymia_

Recurrent Major Depression w/o
Interepisode Full Recovery w/o

Early/Late-onset: _Late_

Answers to Diagnostic Exercise 4

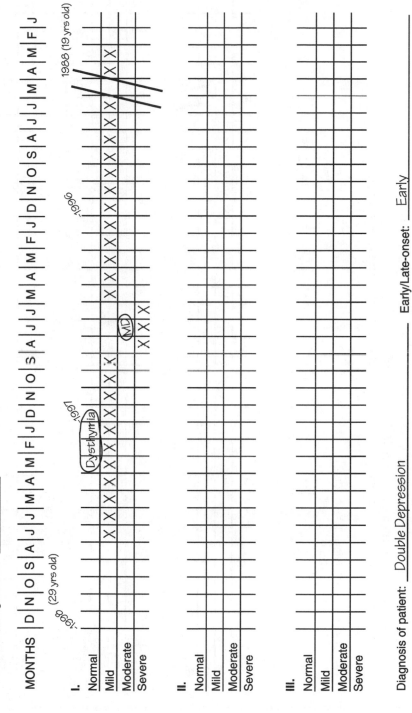

INSTRUCTIONS

1. Work from left to right and mark "X's" under the appropriate months.
2. Start by writing current year; begin rating in current month.
3. Use Timeline I to establish chronic course of present disorder.
4. Use Timelines II and III to plot course over the life span (note "years" as much as possible).

Year of screening interview __1998__

MONTHS | D | N | O | S | A | J | J | M | A | M | F | J | D | N | O | S | A | J | J | M | A | M | F | J | D | N | O | S | A | J | J | M | A | M | F | J

I.

Normal
Mild
Moderate
Severe

II.

Normal
Mild
Moderate
Severe

III.

Normal
Mild
Moderate
Severe

Diagnosis of patient: ___Double Depression___   Early/Late-onset: ___Early___

Answers to Diagnostic Exercise 5

41

INSTRUCTIONS

1. Work from left to right and mark "X's" under the appropriate months.
2. Start by writing current year; begin rating in current month.
3. Use Timeline I to establish chronic course of present disorder.
4. Use Timelines II and III to plot course over the life span (note "years" as much as possible).

Year of screening interview 1997

MONTHS D | N | O | S | A | J | J | M | A | M | F | J | D | N | O | S | A | J | J | M | A | M | F | J | D | N | O | S | A | J | J | M | A | M | F | J

(52 yrs old)

-1997   -1996   -1995   High School
                                       (Early-onset)

I.
Normal
Mild
Moderate
Severe

II.
Normal
Mild
Moderate
Severe

III.
Normal
Mild
Moderate
Severe

Diagnosis of patient: Pure Dysthymia   Early/Late-onset: Early

Answers to Diagnostic Exercise 6

INSTRUCTIONS
1. Work from left to right and mark "X's" under the appropriate months.
2. Start by writing current year; begin rating in current month.
3. Use Timeline I to establish chronic course of present disorder.
4. Use Timelines II and III to plot course over the life span (note "years" as much as possible).

Year of screening interview ___1999___

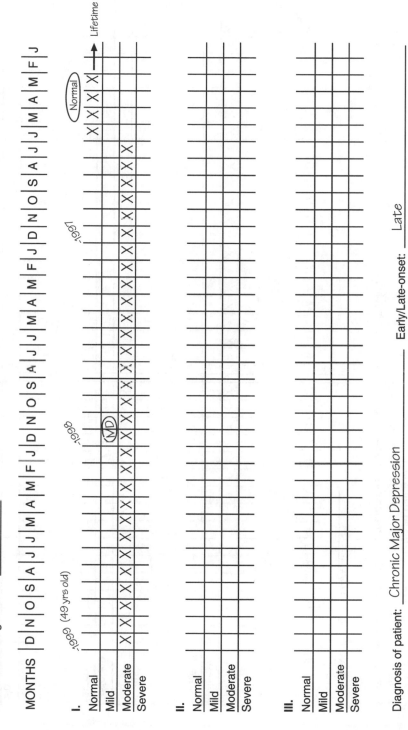

Diagnosis of patient: ___Chronic Major Depression___   Early/Late-onset: ___Late___

Answers to Diagnostic Exercise 7

43

INSTRUCTIONS

1. Work from left to right and mark "X's" under the appropriate months.
2. Start by writing current year; begin rating in current month.
3. Use Timeline I to establish chronic course of present disorder.
4. Use Timelines II and III to plot course over the life span (note "years" as much as possible).

Year of screening interview 1999

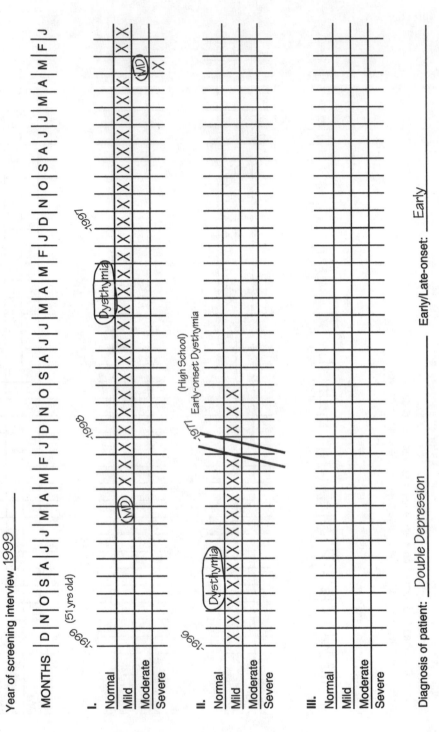

Diagnosis of patient: Double Depression   Early/Late-onset: Early

Answers to Diagnostic Exercise 8

INSTRUCTIONS
1. Work from left to right and mark "X's" under the appropriate months.
2. Start by writing current year; begin rating in current month.
3. Use Timeline I to establish chronic course of present disorder.
4. Use Timelines II and III to plot course over the life span (note "years" as much as possible).

Year of screening interview ___2000___

MONTHS | D | N | O | S | A | J | J | M | A | M | F | J | D | N | O | S | A | J | J | M | A | M | F | J

'2000 (37 yrs old)   '1999   '1998

I.

Normal	
Mild	
Moderate	X X X X X X X X X X X X X X X X X X X X X X X X ⓂⒹ X X X X X X X X X X X X X X X X X X X
Severe	

'1997   '1996

II.

Normal	
Mild	
Moderate	X X X X X X X X X X X X X ⓂⒹ X X X X X X X X X X X X ⒹⓎⓈⓣⓗⓨⓜⓘⓐ X X X X X X X X X X X X X
Severe	X X X X X X X X X X X X

(High School)
Early-onset Dysthymia

III.

Normal	
Mild	
Moderate	
Severe	

Diagnosis of patient: ___Double Depression (Chronic MD with Antecedent Dysthymia)___   Early/Late-onset: ___Early___

Answers to Diagnostic Exercise 9

45

INSTRUCTIONS

1. Work from left to right and mark "X's" under the appropriate months.
2. Start by writing current year; begin rating in current month.
3. Use Timeline I to establish chronic course of present disorder.
4. Use Timelines II and III to plot course over the life span (note "years" as much as possible).

Year of screening interview 1999

MONTHS | D | N | O | S | A | J | J | M | A | M | F | J | D | N | O | S | A | J | J | M | A | M | F | J | D | N | O | S | A | J | J | M | A | M | F | J

I.

	'1999 (31 yrs old)												'1998												'1997											
Normal																																				
Mild																																				
Moderate					X	X	X	X	X	X	X	X	X	X	X	X	X	X	X	X					X	X	X	X	X	X	X	X	X	X	X	X
Severe			X																																	

MD (circled)

Hospitalization

Hospitalization

II.

	'19??																																			
Normal																																				
Mild	X	X		X	X	X	X																													
Moderate																																				
Severe		X	X																																	

Hospitalization (23 yrs old)

MD (circled)

Lifetime →

III.

Normal																																				
Mild																																				
Moderate																																				
Severe																																				

Diagnosis of patient: Recurrent Major Depression w/o Interepisode Full Recovery w/o Antecedent Dysthymia   Early/Late-onset: Late

Answers to Diagnostic Exercise 10

FOUR

Administering Situational Analysis

PART I
Situational Analysis: Elicitation Phase Exercises

The chronically depressed patient's interpersonal behavior imposes a severe behavioral restriction on psychotherapists:

Therapists must avoid assuming a dominant and take-charge interpersonal role with patients.

Dominant therapist behavior is destructive and precludes change with chronically depressed patients. In the text, *Treatment for Chronic Depression*, I describe the dominant, take-charge style as therapeutically lethal. Chronic patients, because of their helpless and hopeless demeanor, interpersonally "pull," "evoke"—and, yes, "demand"—that clinicians do their work for them. It is also easy for therapists to expect very little from these patients, and consequently patients usually initiate very little activity; instead, they wait for therapists to tell them what to do.

The pull for dominance also comes from the chronic patient's interpersonal submissiveness. The reason that dominance is so destructive with this type of patient is because it reinforces and maintains the patient's submissiveness, compliance, and feelings of helplessness.

Significant portions of Part II of the text discuss several strategies to help therapists curtail the dominant style. In particular, Chapters Six and Seven describe the administration of Situational Analysis (SA) within a framework of "Therapist Rules" and "Patient Performance Goals." The rules for SA dictate that the patient, not the clinician, must do the work. The therapist must follow the patient's lead rather than pull or push him/her through the steps of SA. The ultimate performance goals for SA are made explicit to each patient: "*You must learn to do each of the SA steps by yourself and without assistance from the clinician.*"

Interestingly, your training role at this point is similar to that of the beginning psychotherapy patient: You, too, must undertake learning SA from the beginning. Rather than just tell you what to do, I am going to follow you gently with my answers (like I want you to do with your patients), until you learn the SA steps and become more confident in your ability to do the steps by yourself. Another major goal of this chapter is to teach you to discriminate criterion SA performance from substandard performance.

Feedback will be provided after you have completed each exercise. In instances where my feedback is unclear and you still remain confused, please refer to the text (Chapters Six and Seven). The evaluative decisions you will make in the exercises about the patient's performance will be similar to the ones you will have to make when you see actual patients. Chronically depressed patients throw us "difficult SA pitches to hit." The more skilled you become at *recognizing* and *managing* the various difficult pitches you are thrown in the manual, the more likely you will be able to identify your patients' errors and respond effectively.

The SA technique is administered using the Coping Style Questionnaire (CSQ). The patient is given several CSQs at the end of session 2 and instructed to complete one CSQ prior to each therapy session. SA will then be conducted using the homework CSQ. Each step in SA is based on the CSQ format, and during situational analysis, the patient refers frequently to his/her CSQ notes. An example CSQ form is shown in Figure 4.

Patient: _____   Therapist: _____

Date of Situational Event: _____   Date of Therapy Session: _____

Instructions: Select one interpersonal problematic or successful event that has happened to you during the past week and describe it using the format below. Please try to fill out all parts of the questionnaire. Your therapist will assist you in situational analysis during your next therapy session.

Situational Area: Spouse/Partner ____   Children ____   Extended Family ____
Work/School ____   Social ____

Step 1. Describe what happened.

Step 2. Describe your interpretation of what happened. (How did you "read" the situation?)
  1.

  2.

  3.

Step 3. Describe what you did during the situation (what you said/how you said it).

Step 4. Describe how the event came out for you (actual outcome).

Step 5. Describe how you wanted the event to come out for you (desired outcome).

Step 6. Was the desired outcome achieved?   Yes____   No____

FIGURE 4. Coping Survey Questionnaire (CSQ).

As stated above, the goal in this chapter is to teach you to discriminate criterion-level SA performance from substandard performance. The elicitation phase includes 6 steps; parallel learning exercises comprise Part I of this chapter. Each exercise provides opportunities to make criterion evaluations about the adequacy of the patient's performance and, in some instances, the adequacy of your own performance. The exercises start with simple problems and become progressively more difficult.

As in Chapter Three, after completing each exercise, turn to the indicated page for the answers. Again, refer to Chapters Six and Seven in the text whenever you do not understand my feedback.

STEP 1: SITUATIONAL DESCRIPTION

Review

Review the "Therapist Rules for Administering Step 1" in the text (pp. 110–113) and summarized here:

1. Provide a rationale to the patient for Step 1 (text, p. 110).
2. Teach the patient to describe one situational event that has a beginning, an exit or endpoint, and a story in between.
3. Tell the patient that the situation may be either a problematical or a successful event.
4. Teach the patient to describe the event from an "observer" perspective (discourage editorializing or attributing motives [mind reading] to the other person in the situation).
5. At the end, summarize the situational description, using the patient's language (avoid paraphrasing or using your own pet phrases).

Review the "Patient Performance Goal for Step 1" in the text (p. 113) and summarized here:

1. Describe a situational event in an objective and succinct manner.

Sample Criterion Situational Description

"I had an argument with my wife last night over who would pay the bills this month. We started counting back to see how many times she and I had done it this year. Then she said I didn't carry my weight with the chores around the house. I answered her in kind with a comment like, 'Who earns the most money?' With that remark, both of us looked at each other and laughed. Then I shifted the focus to whose schedule would allow the most time to pay the bills. We decided that mine was the most flexible, so I said I would pay the bills. We resolved a difficult argument and solved the problem. The situation ended when we decided that I would pay the bills."

Comment: The description has a clear beginning point, clear exit/endpoint, a continuous story in between, and the description is told in "observer terminology" that gives the therapist a good understanding of the interaction between the patient and his wife.

Exercises

1. Answer the questions found at the end of each exercise. Try to identify the patient performance errors or the lack thereof.
2. If errors exist in the situational description, describe each error in the space provided.
3. After completing each exercise, *check your evaluation of the patient's performance with the criterion answers on pp. 60 64.*

Situational Description 1

"I get rejected by people all the time. Nothing ever works out for me."

Answer each question below:

1. Does the description have a clear beginning point? (Yes/No)
2. Does the description have a clear exit or endpoint? (Yes/No)
3. Does the description have a continuous story in between the beginning and exit or endpoint? (Yes/No)
4. Is the description told from an observer (behavioral language) perspective? (Yes/No)
5. List briefly what problem(s) are contained in the above situational description (refer to the Therapist Rules and Patient Performance Goal in text, pp. 110–113): _____

   _____

   _____

   _____

   _____

Check your work with the criterion answers on p. 60.

Situational Description 2

"I've had a really boring week and nothing has gone the way I wanted it to."

Answer each question below:

1. Does the description have a clear beginning point? (Yes/No)
2. Does the description have a clear exit or endpoint? (Yes/No)
3. Does the description have a continuous story in between the beginning and exit or endpoint? (Yes/No)
4. Is the description told from an observer (behavioral language) perspective? (Yes/No)
5. List briefly what problem(s) are contained in the above situational description:_____

   _____

   _____

   _____

   _____

Check your work with the criterion answers on p. 60.

Situational Description 3

"My girlfriend and I went out on Monday evening, had dinner together on Tuesday, and she stayed over at my house Wednesday night. It's been a great week."

Answer each question below:

1. Does the description have a clear beginning point? (Yes/No)
2. Does the description have a clear exit or endpoint? (Yes/No)
3. Does the description have a continuous story in between the beginning and exit or endpoint? (Yes/No)
4. Is the description told from an observer (behavioral language) perspective? (Yes/No)
5. List briefly what problem(s) are contained in the above situational description:_____

_____

_____

_____

_____

Check your work with the criterion answers on p. 60.

Situational Description 4

"My situation happened last week. I met friends at a restaurant and the dinner was enjoyable. Everyone ate a lot and felt good."

Answer each question below:

1. Does the description have a clear beginning point? (Yes/No)
2. Does the description have a clear exit or endpoint? (Yes/No)
3. Does the description have a continuous story in between the beginning and exit or endpoint? (Yes/No)
4. Is the description told from an observer (behavioral language) perspective? (Yes/No)
5. List briefly what problem(s) are contained in the above situational description:_____

_____

_____

_____

_____

Check your work with the criterion answers on p. 60.

Situational Description 5

"I went to the grocery story to buy a pound of sugar. Bought it and returned home."

Answer each question below:

1. Does the description have a clear beginning point? (Yes/No)
2. Does the description have a clear exit or endpoint? (Yes/No)
3. Does the description have a continuous story in between the beginning and exit or endpoint? (Yes/No)
4. Is the description told from an observer (behavioral language) perspective? (Yes/No)
5. List briefly what problem(s) are contained in the above situational description:_____

_____

_____

_____

_____

Check your work with the criterion answers on pp. 60–61.

Situational Description 6

"Phoned my son at college last Sunday and we talked for about 15 minutes. Neither one of us said very much to each other. Then I told him goodbye and hung up."

Answer each question below:

1. Does the description have a clear beginning point? (Yes/No)
2. Does the description have a clear exit or endpoint? (Yes/No)
3. Does the description have a continuous story in between the beginning and exit or endpoint? (Yes/No)
4. Is the description told from an observer (behavioral language) perspective? (Yes/No)
5. List briefly what problem(s) are contained in the above situational description: _____

_____

_____

_____

_____

Check your work with the criterion answers on p. 61.

Situational Description 7

"Last night I finally told my roommate how I felt about his leaving his clothes all over our apartment. Said to him that I didn't like it and that I wanted him to start picking up his stuff. He said he would and then he apologized for his sloppiness. God, did that feel really good."

Answer each question below:

1. Does the description have a clear beginning point? (Yes/No)
2. Does the description have a clear exit or endpoint? (Yes/No)

3. Does the description have a continuous story in between the beginning and exit or endpoint? (Yes/No)
4. Is the description told from an observer (behavioral language) perspective? (Yes/No)
5. List briefly what problem(s) are contained in the above situational description: _____

_____

_____

_____

_____

Check your work with the criterion answers on p. 61.

Situational Description 8

"I want to feel confident about what I do. Like when I have to make a talk in front of the office staff. I always feel afraid that I will mess up. I just wish I could feel confident. I think about being in front of a group, and I get scared to death."

Answer each question below:

1. Does the description have a clear beginning point? (Yes/No)
2. Does the description have a clear exit or endpoint? (Yes/No)
3. Does the description have a continuous story in between the beginning and the exit or endpoint? (Yes/No)
4. Is the description told from an observer (behavioral language) perspective? (Yes/No)
5. List briefly what problem(s) are contained in the above situational description: _____

_____

_____

_____

_____

Check your work with the criterion answers on p. 61.

Situational Description 9

"The week has been a bummer. Nothing has worked out for me. Had an argument with my office mate, my boss and I had a run-in, my girlfriend got angry with me. I was glad when Friday rolled around, and it was quitting time. I got out of the office in a hurry and went to a bar."

Answer each question below:

1. Does the description have a clear beginning point? (Yes/No)
2. Does the description have a clear exit or endpoint? (Yes/No)
3. Does the description have a continuous story in between the beginning and exit or endpoint? (Yes/No)

4. Is the description told from an observer (behavioral language) perspective? (Yes/No)
5. List briefly what problem(s) are contained in the above situational description: _____

_____

_____

_____

_____

Check your work with the criterion answers on pp. 61–62.

Situational Description 10

"Wanted to take my broken lawn mower to the Sears repair shop on Saturday. Bought some gas for the car on the way and delivered the mower to Sears and left it. Got back to the house about an hour later."

Answer each question below:

1. Does the description have a clear beginning point? (Yes/No)
2. Does the description have a clear exit or endpoint? (Yes/No)
3. Does the description have a continuous story in between the beginning and exit or endpoint? (Yes/No)
4. Is the description told from an observer (behavioral language) perspective? (Yes/No)
5. List briefly what problem(s) are contained in the above situational description: _____

_____

_____

_____

_____

Check your work with the criterion answers on p. 62.

Situational Description 11

"I was going to meet a male friend for lunch at a restaurant, and I wore my best skirt and matching blouse. My hair was fixed just the way I like it. I put on a necklace and earrings that go well with the outfit and walked from my office to the restaurant. I was a little early so I decided to walk down a side street and window shop. Spent about 15 minutes looking at the merchandise. The dresses were bright spring colors, and I really liked the shoes on display, and there was one antique store that had some end tables that are like the ones I have in my apartment. I saw a neighbor, and he and I talked about the latest neighborhood gossip. He told me he's separated from his wife—he even hinted that he would like to go out with me. I like him but have never found him attractive. If he ever asked me out, I'd have to tell him something. Not sure what I would say. Guess I'd think of something. Told him goodbye and then ran into my rabbi. He and I talked about the synagogue. He inquired where I had been the past few weeks. Wasn't sure what to say to him, so I made some excuse. I finally got to the restaurant to meet my friend. Long lunch, eh!"

Answer each question below:

1. Does the description have a clear beginning point? (Yes/No)
2. Does the description have a clear exit or endpoint? (Yes/No)
3. Does the description have a continuous story in between the beginning and exit or endpoint? (Yes/No)
4. Is the description told from an observer (behavioral language) perspective? (Yes/No)
5. List briefly what problem(s) are contained in the above situational description: _____

_____

_____

_____

_____

Check your work with the criterion answers on p. 62.

Situational Description 12

"Nothing of any significance happened to me this week. I just talked to several people, and they were okay."

Answer each question below:

1. Does the description have a clear beginning point? (Yes/No)
2. Does the description have a clear exit or endpoint? (Yes/No)
3. Does the description have a continuous story in between the beginning and exit or endpoint? (Yes/No)
4. Is the description told from an observer (behavioral language) perspective? (Yes/No)
5. List briefly what problem(s) are contained in the above situational description: _____

_____

_____

_____

_____

Check your work with the criterion answers on p. 62.

Situational Description 13

"I wanted him to ask me out. I've waited all day beginning at 8:00 A.M. for him to call me. He never did and I went to bed about 10:00 P.M. Guess he thinks I'm a loser."

Answer each question below:

1. Does the description have a clear beginning point? (Yes/No)
2. Does the description have a clear exit or endpoint? (Yes/No)
3. Does the description have a continuous story in between the beginning and exit or endpoint? (Yes/No)

4. Is the description told from an observer (behavioral language) perspective? (Yes/No)
5. List briefly what problem(s) are contained in the above situational description: _____

_____

_____

_____

_____

Check your work with the criterion answers on pp. 62–63.

Situational Description 14

"My wife and I were eating supper last night. Our son had gone to a movie. We got into another argument over something our son had done the day before. She told me how she had reacted to him and I called her 'stupid.' She got mad, as usual. I don't know why we fight so much. Everything we talk about ends up in a fight. Both of us walked away from the table not speaking to each other."

Answer each question below:

1. Does the description have a clear beginning point? (Yes/No)
2. Does the description have a clear exit or endpoint? (Yes/No)
3. Does the description have a continuous story in between the beginning and exit or endpoint? (Yes/No)
4. Is the description told from an observer (behavioral language) perspective? (Yes/No)
5. List briefly what problem(s) are contained in the above situational description: _____

_____

_____

_____

_____

Check your work with the criterion answers on p. 63.

Situational Description 15

"I'm always screwing up what I try to do. This situation is just like all the rest. I end up saying something stupid. Then the other person takes it the wrong way, and I end up feeling like *I've done it again.*"

Answer each question below:

1. Does the description have a clear beginning point? (Yes/No)
2. Does the description have a clear exit or endpoint? (Yes/No)
3. Does the description have a continuous story in between the beginning and exit or endpoint? (Yes/No)
4. Is the description told from an observer (behavioral language) perspective? (Yes/No)

5. List briefly what problem(s) are contained in the above situational description: _____

_____

_____

_____

_____

Check your work with the criterion answers on p. 63.

Situational Description 16

"My boyfriend came over to the house last night, and we watched TV. He wanted me to go to bed with him, but I wasn't in the mood. He started calling me names. Told me what a loser I was. I didn't say anything to defend myself. I just took his verbal abuse in silence. Finally, he told me he was leaving, and he did. He didn't even say goodnight."

Answer each question below:

1. Does the description have a clear beginning point? (Yes/No)
2. Does the description have a clear exit or endpoint? (Yes/No)
3. Does the description have a continuous story in between the beginning and exit or endpoint? (Yes/No)
4. Is the description told from an observer (behavioral language) perspective? (Yes/No)
5. List briefly what problem(s) are contained in the above situational description: _____

_____

_____

_____

_____

Check your work with the criterion answers on p. 63.

Situational Description 17

"I met an old friend on campus today that I haven't seen in a year. We had a serious disagreement the last time we were together, even got mad at each other, and both of us had said some unkind things to one another. She was being extra nice today. I think her niceness was stemming from her still being angry with me. I just knew she was still mad. We talked, then said goodbye. I just know that she is still angry with me."

Answer each question below:

1. Does the description have a clear beginning point? (Yes/No)
2. Does the description have a clear exit or endpoint? (Yes/No)
3. Does the description have a continuous story in between the beginning and exit or endpoint? (Yes/No)
4. Is the description told from an observer(behavioral language) perspective? (Yes/No)

5. List briefly what problem(s) are contained in the above situational description: _____

_____

_____

_____

_____

Check your work with the criterion answers on pp. 63–64.

Situational Description 18

"Wednesday, my boss and I talked. Given his negative comments about my project work, I knew he thought that I had done a sloppy job with the project he had given me to complete. He made several suggestions about improving my work and how I might tighten up the report. I felt he was just being overly polite. What he really wanted to say was that I had done a poor job. When he finished giving me feedback, I left his office."

Answer each question below:

1. Does the description have a clear beginning point? (Yes/No)
2. Does the description have a clear exit or endpoint? (Yes/No)
3. Does the description have a continuous story in between the beginning and exit or endpoint? (Yes/No)
4. Is the description told from an observer (behavioral language) perspective? (Yes/No)
5. List briefly what problem(s) are contained in the above situational description: _____

_____

_____

_____

_____

Check your work with the criterion answers on p. 64.

Situational Description 19

"Friday afternoon my colleague and I were talking about how we might solve a serious problem concerning an office policy that has been a bone of contention for everyone. He took a view that was diametrically opposed to mine. He usually comes at me this way about anything we talk about. We got into an argument again and never could agree on the best way to address the office policy. Finally, both of us agreed that we were wasting time talking about the issue. He went his way and I went mine."

Answer each question below:

1. Does the description have a clear beginning point? (Yes/No)
2. Does the description have a clear exit or endpoint? (Yes/No)

3. Does the description have a continuous story in between the beginning and exit or endpoint? (Yes/No)
4. Is the description told from an observer (behavioral language) perspective? (Yes/No)
5. List briefly what problem(s) are contained in the above situational description: _____

_____

_____

_____

_____

Check your work with the criterion answers on p. 64.

Situational Description 20

"I wanted a package wrapped at the store Saturday before I went to a birthday party for my girlfriend. The gift wrap department was about to close when I took the ticket designating my turn in the waiting line. I asked one of the wrappers if she could do it for me—said I was going to a party, and I couldn't go without getting the box wrapped. Looked her right in the eye when I asked her. She nodded and told me to wait around, and she would do it for me. She wrapped the gift, and it looked beautiful. I tipped her $5 and went to the party."

Answer each question below:

1. Does the description have a clear beginning point? (Yes/No)
2. Does the description have a clear exit or endpoint? (Yes/No)
3. Does the description have a continuous story in between the beginning and the exit or endpoint? (Yes/No)
4. Is the description told from an observer (behavioral language) perspective? (Yes/No)
5. List briefly what problem(s) are contained in the above situational description: _____

_____

_____

_____

_____

Check your work with the criterion answers on p. 64.

Criterion Answers for Step 1 Elicitation Exercises

Situational Description 1

1. No.
2. No.
3. No.
4. No.
5. The event is not pinpointed in time. No story is told. The exit/endpoint event is not specified. The observer perspective is not achieved.

Situational Description 2

1. No.
2. No.
3. No.
4. No.
5. The event is not pinpointed in time. No story is told. No exit/endpoint is specified. The observer perspective is not achieved.

Situational Description 3

1. No.
2. No.
3. No.
4. No.
5. The event is not pinpointed in time. No story is told. No exit/endpoint is specified. The observer perspective is not achieved.

Situational Description 4

1. No.
2. No.
3. No.
4. No.
5. The event is indirectly but inadequately pinpointed in time. No story is told. No exit/endpoint is specified. The observer perspective is not achieved.

Situational Description 5

1. Yes. However, the description is too global and requires the therapist to infer too much.
2. Yes.
3. Yes. [There are the "skeletal" beginnings of a story, but more elaboration is needed.]
4. No.

5. Because the storyline is skeletal, the description gives the clinician nothing interpersonal with which to work. Patients who construct such stories usually avoid interpersonal encounters. The real issue is, Why the avoidance?

Situational Description 6

1. Yes.
2. Yes.
3. No. [There is only a skeletal report of conversation that provides no information concerning the exchange between the father and his son.]
4. Yes.
5. Patient must begin to describe situations in more specific detail so that the therapist has a clearer idea of what happened between the two interactants. For example: Did the father try to engage his son in conversation? Did the son respond or initiate conversation, etc.?

Situational Description 7

1. Yes.
2. Yes.
3. Yes.
4. Yes. [The subjective statement at the end is acceptable because we have a clear idea of what happened and how the situation ended.]
5. This situational description is acceptable.

Situational Description 8

1. No.
2. No.
3. No.
4. No.
5. The event is not pinpointed in time. No story is told. No exit/endpoint is specified. The observer perspective is not achieved.

Situational Description 9

1. No.
2. Yes. [But the exit/endpoint ends with no content or continuous story preceding it. The patient has not yet learned to select one "slice-of-time" and describe it for the situation.]
3. No. [We have a collage of several events that are patched together.]
4. Yes. [Patient succeeds here but still must learn to select one of the events and focus on this alone.]

5. The event is not pinpointed in time. No continuous story is told. The exit/endpoint is specified, but the lack of internal continuity makes the endpoint useless. The observer perspective is achieved—but, again, it is useless because of the lack of internal consistency.

Situational Description 10

1. Yes. [But paucity of information about the interpersonal encounter makes the description useless.]
2. Yes. [Again, the skeletal description is not conducive for effective SA work.]
3. Yes. [Same comment as above.]
4. Yes. [Same comment as above.]
5. The marked and consistent absence of interpersonal involvement is characteristic of schizoid patients or other patients who actively avoid interacting with other people.

Situational Description 11

1. Yes.
2. Yes.
3. No. [The story is filled with subevents that detract from the encounter with the male at the restaurant. There is too much information in the description. If the story had been told in the following sequence, we would have had a story we could work with: Patient went to a restaurant → description of what happened between the patient and man during lunch → the encounter ended, and the patient left the restaurant.]
4. No. [Personal editorializing continues throughout the situational description.]
5. There is no story evident, even though the event is pinpointed in time. The observer focus is not achieved. Patient must learn to attend to the relevant details of the situation.

Situational Description 12

1. No.
2. No.
3. No.
4. No.
5. Situational pinpointing is absent and the lack of focus means that the patient is unable to select one specific slice-of-time to use for a description.

Situational Description 13

1. Yes.
2. Yes.
3. No. [This example is instructive because it shows us what to avoid in SA. Do not conduct an SA on something that hasn't happened. Why? Because everything will

be speculative—a perspective you want to help patients avoid. Patients must be taught to ground themselves in real-world events and not the non-events of their imagination.]

4. No.
5. The focus is on a non-event—on something that hasn't happened.

Situational Description 14

1. Yes.
2. Yes.
3. Yes.
4. Yes.
5. All the criterion requirements are met in this description. The only problem is the parsimony of the content. The patient will have to learn to elaborate more in future descriptions so that the clinician will have a clearer picture of what actually happened. But this is a good start.

Situational Description 15

1. No.
2. No.
3. No. [The description is vague and overly global. It is not focused on behavioral specifics such as, "He said this, I said that, then this happened."]
4. No. [Considerable "mind-reading" of the other person is present. The real problem is that we know nothing about the other interactant. Teach patients to stick to details of the actual events.]
5. The patient tries to focus on a slice-of-time. However, the attempt is not successful, and the description is inadequate in every respect.

Situational Description 16

1. Yes.
2. Yes.
3. Yes.
4. Yes.
5. This is an adequate situational description that can be used for SA. The beginning and endpoint are firmly set, and the story in between provides a useable description of the interaction. The story is also told from an acceptable observer perspective.

Situational Description 17

1. Yes.
2. Yes.
3. Yes.

4. Yes/no. [The patient must learn to describe the situation without editorializing or mind-reading. These are features of the description that can be easily extinguished.]
5. Other than the editorializing/mind-reading, this is an adequate description that can be used for SA.

Situational Description 18

1. Yes.
2. Yes.
3. Yes/no. [The patient is editorializing as well as mind-reading. Teach patients to stick with the facts, not inferences. This description is similar to the preceding one in that both patients must learn to describe an event while remaining in an observer mode.]
4. No. [Learning to describe the situation as an observer is the major task here.]
5. Extinguish the embellishments that are added to an otherwise acceptable situational description.

Situational Description 19

1. Yes. [Excellent beginning.]
2. Yes. [Excellent exit/endpoint.]
3. Yes. [Excellent story in between.]
4. Yes. [Observer perspective achieved throughout; no editorializing or mind-reading.]
5. There are no problems with this acceptable situational description.

Situational Description 20

1. Yes. [Excellent beginning.]
2. Yes. [Excellent exit/endpoint.]
3. Yes. [Excellent story in between.]
4. Yes. [Observer perspective achieved throughout; no editorializing or mind-reading.]
5. There are no problems with this acceptable situational description.

STEP 2: SITUATIONAL INTERPRETATIONS

Review

Review the "Therapist Rules for Administering Step 2" in the text (pp. 115–122) and summarized here:

1. Provide a rationale to the patient for Step 2 (text, p. 115).
2. Teach the patient to construct one declarative sentence for each interpretation (e.g., "It meant that . . . ").
3. Let the patient do the work.
4. Restate each interpretation using the patient's language.
5. The clinician must understand every word in the interpretation and ask for clarification in instances where the meaning of a word(s) is unclear.
6. Limit the number of interpretations to three or four.
7. Summarize the entire list at the end of the step, using the patient's language.
8. Each interpretation must be *relevant* and *accurate* and describe what is happening in the situation. [*Note*: In actual SA administration, this rule applies only during the remediation phase of SA. It is stated here because you will be asked to construct interpretations below that meet the *relevancy* and *accuracy* criteria.]

Reminder: Since many psychotherapists have been trained in Beck's cognitive therapy (CT), a reminder is provided to help trainees discriminate between the role cognitive beliefs, attitudes, and automatic thoughts play in CT versus the role cognitive interpretations play in Situational Analysis. In CT, cognitive constructs are assessed in terms of the degree to which they accurately appraise reality. In CT, a realistic appraisal or cognition is one that validly assesses reality.

The role of the cognitive interpretation in SA is a functional one; that is, it either contributes, or does not contribute, to the attainment of the desired outcome. In order to contribute functionally to the achievement of the desired outcome, a cognitive interpretation must two criteria: (1) it must be firmly grounded in the situational event (*relevance*); and (2) it must accurately describe *what* is happening in the interpersonal event (*accuracy*).

Review the "Patient Performance Goal for Step 2" in the text (p. 122) and summarized here:

1. Patient learns to construct relevant and accurate interpretations without assistance from the clinician.

Sample Criterion Situational Interpretations

SITUATIONAL DESCRIPTION

"I drove my roommate to our university classes yesterday—we live off campus. He and I are very competitive with each other, and we had gotten into an argument the night before over who was the better pitcher for the Atlanta Braves, Greg Maddox or Tom Glavine. I thought Maddox was, and he argued that I was wrong, it was Glavine. The argument got pretty hot, and finally I said to him, 'You are stupid and don't know a thing about baseball.' He got mad at me and pretty much said the same thing to me. We didn't speak to each other the rest of the evening. On the way to school, I told him that my comment had been stupid and that I was sorry I said what I did. He apologized to me for what he said. We got to school and went our separate ways."

INTERPRETATIONS

1. "I really disagree with the position my roommate is taking."
2. "Greg Maddox has no peers when it comes to pitching."
3. "I'm really mad."
4. "I must apologize for my comment."

Comment: Interpretations 1–3 meet the criteria of relevancy (anchored temporally in the situation) and accuracy (describe what is going on in the situation). Interpretation 4 is an *action interpretation* that usually leads to assertive behavior.

Exercises

Following are 10 situational interpretation exercises. For each:

1. Read the situational description and construct three or four relevant and accurate interpretations. [*Note:* You will be taking the role of the patient. It is important to note that the interpretations you obtain from patients during Step 2 will more than likely have to be revised/reworked during the remediation phase (see text, pp. 143–157). However, the goal here is to help you learn to construct *relevant* and *accurate* interpretations. This will help you recognize criterion-level interpretations when you begin eliciting interpretations from patients.]
2. Spaces are provided in each exercise for four interpretations. You do *not* have to construct four interpretations for each exercise, and do not construct more than four.
3. Check your interpretations for each exercise with the criterion answers on pp. 73–74. [*Note:* You may construct interpretational sentences that differ somewhat from my criterion interpretations. If your interpretations meet the relevancy and accuracy criteria, then they are correct.]

Situational Interpretations 1

"I had a bad encounter with my husband last night. I began the conversation trying to tell him that he had overdrawn our checking account again. He said, 'Oh no! You're going to lay into me again!' I said that since he never records the checks he writes, our balance is always unknown. He became real angry and yelled at me, saying that from now on I'm going to have to do all the grocery shopping because he won't. I didn't reply or say anything else. The conversation ended with us not speaking to each other."

a. Write out your interpretations:

1. _____
2. _____
3. _____
4. _____

b. *Check your interpretations with the criterion interpretations found on p. 73. How did your* interpretations compare with the criterion interpretations? Pinpoint any differences on the following lines.

_____

_____

_____

_____

FEEDBACK QUESTIONS

- Did you mind-read the husband's motives [always an inaccurate interpretation: see text, p. 122]? (Yes/No)
- Did any of your interpretations become global (e.g., "We always end up fighting this way" etc.) [inaccurate interpretation: see text, pp. 117–118, 122]? (Yes/No)

Situational Interpretations 2

"Rob asked me out last night, and he wanted me to decide on the movie. I told him that I didn't care what we saw. He refused to make the decision and just got mad and pouted because I wouldn't make the decision. We didn't go to a movie. We stopped in at a McDonald's for coffee. He told me that I had ruined the evening for him. We decided to leave McDonald's, and we left the coffee on the table. We drove home, and he let me out in the driveway. I walked into the house alone and was furious with him."

a. Write out your interpretations:

1. _____
2. _____
3. _____
4. _____

b. *Check your interpretations with the criterion interpretations on p. 73. How did your inter*pretations compare with the criterion interpretations? Pinpoint any differences on the following lines.

_____

_____

_____

_____

FEEDBACK QUESTIONS

- Did you mind-read the boyfriend's motives/behaviors? (Yes/No)
- Were any of your interpretations global? (Yes/No)
- Did your interpretations describe what was taking place in the situation? (Yes/No)

Situational Interpretations 3

"The work supervisor called me into her office on Tuesday. The meeting was my first 6-month evaluation with the company. My supervisor gave me "average" ratings in all the work categories. I thought I had done much better in several categories and told her so. I had worked late many nights, initiated several projects on my own, and had given my colleagues help on numerous occasions. My supervisor knew nothing about these things, and she told me I should have let her know. She also said that she would not change her original evaluation of my work. I signed the evaluation and left her office."

a. Write out your interpretations:

1. _____
2. _____
3. _____
4. _____

b. *Check your interpretations with the criterion interpretations on p. 73.* How did your interpretations compare with the criterion interpretations? Pinpoint any differences on the following lines.

_____
_____
_____
_____

Situational Interpretations 4

"I went into a 7-Eleven store to buy some milk. I brought the milk to the check-out line and waited. I was about fifth in line. The cashier let three people in line ahead of me. I didn't say anything, just waited my turn. When the cashier finally took my money, he never asked me if I wanted a bag for the gallon jug. I picked up the change and the milk and left the store."

a. Write out your interpretations:

1. _____
2. _____
3. _____
4. _____

b. *Check your interpretations with the criterion interpretations on p. 73.* How did your interpretations compare with the criterion interpretations? Pinpoint any differences on the following lines.

_____

_____

_____

_____

FEEDBACK QUESTIONS

Are you still having difficulty? If so, identify the difficulty: _____

_____

_____

Note: If you are still having difficulty, reread Chapter Six (pp. 115–122) in the text. Remember, the functions of cognitive interpretations in CBASP are to keep patients grounded in the situation as well as to help them accurately appraise what is actually happening. Grounding and accurate appraisal are prerequisites for obtaining the desired outcome.

Situational Interpretations 5

"I answered a telemarketing call the other evening during supper. A stockbroker from New York called me. I tried to get off the phone politely, but he kept asking me about my investments. I told him several stocks I had invested in. He asked me what kind of annual dividends I was getting, and I told him. He told me that he could make me more money. I said I wasn't interested in changing my portfolio at this time. He wouldn't stop talking to me. I couldn't get him to stop. Finally, he told me I was a stupid investor and he hung up. I got really depressed and down on myself after I hung up the phone."

a. Write out your interpretations:

1. _____

2. _____

3. _____

4. _____

b. *Check your interpretations with the criterion interpretations on p. 73.* How did your interpretations compare with the criterion interpretations? Pinpoint any differences on the following lines.

_____

_____

_____

_____

FEEDBACK QUESTIONS

- Are you having difficulty with staying grounded in the situation [relevant interpretations]? (Yes/No)
- Are you having difficulty accurately appraising what is going on [accurate interpretations]? (Yes/No)

If you answered yes to one or both questions, review Table 6.2 (p. 118) and Table 6.3 (p. 122) in the text.

Situational Interpretations 6

"I was drinking beer the other night with a friend. We were in a bar where I go quite often. He and I always argue about everything. Tonight was no exception. He is a conservative Republican, and he thinks George W. Bush walks on water—no gun control, pro-life, the whole nine yards. I can't stand Bush, and I told him so. We kept disagreeing over everything and, finally, both of us agreed that it was time to head for home. He never did agree with anything I said the entire night. We told each other goodbye and went our separate ways."

a. Write out your interpretations:

1. _____
2. _____
3. _____
4. _____

b. *Check your interpretations with the criterion interpretations on p. 73.* How did your interpretations compare with the criterion interpretations? Pinpoint any differences on the following lines.

_____
_____
_____
_____

Situational Interpretations 7

"My family and I visited my parents on Christmas morning. This is the time we open packages that have been put under the Christmas tree. My mother made each of my three children sit in a certain place and unwrap their packages without tearing the wrapping paper. When they tore the paper too much, she fussed at them about being wasteful. Then she made each one throw away all the trash in a large trash basket. She didn't want any trash left on the floor. I finally got angry and told her that her routines were silly and took all the fun out of Christmas. I also said that if she didn't stop fussing at the children, we would leave. She didn't say another word to the children about the way they opened their presents. The rest of the morning ended up all right."

a. Write out your interpretations:

1. _____
2. _____
3. _____
4. _____

b. *Check your interpretations with the criterion interpretations on p. 74.* How did your interpretations compare with the criterion interpretations? Pinpoint any differences on the following lines.

_____

_____

_____

_____

Situational Interpretations 8

"My 22-year-old son called me October 15 from Denver and said he needed some money to make it to the end of the month. He's a senior in college. I asked him what he had done with the monthly check we sent him on the first of the month. He said he had spent it. He had been in a poker game and lost badly. I became angry, started cursing, and told him he was irresponsible. Then I started to feel guilty and finally asked how much he needed. He said $500 would do it. I told him I would put the check in the mail today. I got off the phone and was furious—then I got depressed."

a. Write out your interpretations:

1. _____
2. _____
3. _____
4. _____

b. *Check your interpretations with the criterion interpretations on p. 74.* How did your interpretations compare with the criterion interpretations? Pinpoint any differences on the following lines.

_____

_____

_____

_____

Situational Interpretations 9

"I went to Kmart yesterday and ended up with a huge basket of things I wanted to purchase. I waited in line for 15 minutes and finally got up to the cashier. When I got to my car with all the bags, I pulled out the sales ticket and saw that I had been overcharged on several items. One item was a vaseline lip balm container that cost $1.19. I had been charged

$11.95 for the item. I decided not to go back to the store and wait in line again. Driving out of the parking lot, I felt like a real wimp."

a. Write out your interpretations:

1. _____

2. _____

3. _____

4. _____

b. *Check your interpretations with the criterion interpretations on p. 74.* How did your interpretations compare with the criterion interpretations? Pinpoint any differences on the following lines.

_____

_____

_____

_____

Situational Interpretations 10

"My work supervisor gives me nothing but negative feedback. Today he did it again. I had worked hard to put together the display that I took to him to review before I presented it to the board. I thought my work was excellent. I was proud to show it to him. He looked it over and told me that one particular detail was wrong. He also said that I had left out another small detail that I needed to include. He told me to make these corrections before he would pass on it. I left his office feeling that my work was bad. I went back to my office to correct the display errors."

a. Write out your interpretations:

1. _____

2. _____

3. _____

4. _____

b. *Check your interpretations with the criterion interpretations on p. 74.* How did your interpretations compare with the criterion interpretations? Pinpoint any differences on the following lines.

_____

_____

_____

_____

Criterion Answers for Step 2 Elicitation Exercises

Situational Interpretations 1

1. "My husband has overdrawn our account because of his refusal to stub the checks."
2. "My husband is angry."
3. "He won't talk with me about the checkbook problem."

Situational Interpretations 2

1. "Rob wants me to make the decision about what movie to see."
2. "I don't care what we see."
3. "He is angry with me, and he is acting like a spoiled child."

Situational Interpretations 3

1. "I think my evaluations are unduly low."
2. "I never let my supervisor know about all the things I was doing."
3. "I must let her know what I'm doing before the next evaluation [action interpretation]."

Note: See text, pp. 152–153, for an explanation of an "action interpretation" and the role it plays in SA. Action interpretations are necessary to mobilize/prompt assertive behavior appropriate to the situation. The patient must first recognize that assertive behavior is needed to modify a negative state of affairs or to nudge a situation in a desirable direction and then behave accordingly. The assertive behavior can take a verbal and/or nonverbal form.

Situational Interpretations 4

1. "The cashier has let people in ahead of me."
2. "The cashier isn't voluntarily putting the items in a bag."

Situational Interpretations 5

1. "I don't want to talk with this broker."
2. "I disclosed several of my stocks."
3. "I don't want to discuss this further."
4. "He is a rude person."

Situational Interpretations 6

1. "We are arguing again."
2. "I can't stand Bush and what he stands for."
3. "We haven't agreed on anything tonight."

Situational Interpretations 7

1. "It's Christmas morning at home."
2. "My mother is being too controlling with my kids."
3. "I've got to tell her to back off and ease up [this is an action interpretation]."
4. "She backed off and eased up somewhat."

Situational Interpretations 8

1. "My son wants more money."
2. "He spent the previous money playing poker."
3. "He uses my money irresponsibly."
4. "I decided to send him another $500."

Situational Interpretations 9

1. "I've been overcharged."
2. "The lip balm item is grossly overcharged."
3. "I don't want to go back and wait in line again."

Situational Interpretations 10

1. "I got more negative feedback from my supervisor today."
2. "He is missing the 'big picture' here because of attending only to small details."
3. "He wants corrections made before he'll sign off on the project.

Final Remarks about the Step 2 Exercises

The interpretation exercises should give you a clearer understanding of the role played by *relevant*, *accurate*, and *action* interpretations in SA. Interpretations denote a "reading" of what is going on during the event, and in the case of the action read, of what must be done to move the situation in a desirable direction. Said another way, interpretations identify what is actually happening and do not make subjective judgments or qualitative attributions about what is happening (i.e., the goodness, badness, effectiveness, ineffectiveness, adequacy, inadequacy, of the events). Step 2 teaches patients to be "present-focused" throughout an interaction, to be attentive to the moment-to-moment interpersonal fluctuations, and to respond appropriately. Making relevant and accurate interpretations anchors the patient in the present moment.

There is one important aspect of Step 2 construction and evaluation that is not covered in the above exercises, but which you will learn about in the CBASP workshops. Interpretational adequacy depends not only on the relevancy and accuracy of a read but also on whether the read helps the patient obtain what he/she wants in the situation—the desired outcome, or DO. Some CBASP clinicians feel that the most effective interpretations are those that contribute directly to DO attainment. At this point, I am more interested in your acquiring the ability to construct relevant and accurate interpretations. Later you will learn how to help patients evaluate the extent to which their relevant and accurate interpretations contribute (or not) to DO attainment.

I must make one final point about interpretation construction before moving on to Step 3 of SA. The point will become much clearer when we describe Step 2 of the remediation phase and you learn how to revise noncriterion interpretations. CBASP *never* disengages an interpretation from its situational moorings, or considers its adequacy apart from the "actual outcome" (AO)—the consequences of behavior. If we disconnected Step 2 from the situational context as well as from the AO and considered the validity of a particular read apart from the actual situation (as is done in CT; Beck, Rush, Shaw, & Emery, 1979), we would be disengaging cognitive behavior from the consequences it produces. I have worked with many excellent psychotherapists who have been well-trained in the CT tradition. When they first administer CBASP, CT therapists naturally tend to disconnect cognitive interpretations from the AO by viewing Step 2 from the CT perspective. The reason CBASP places so much importance on the way people interpret events is because these situational interpretations lead directly to environmental consequences (the AO). Whenever we view interpretations as an independent construct and conceptualize them as a dysfunctional belief, attitude, or automatic thought (Beck et al., 1979), we risk losing the situational consequences of cognitive behavior.

STEP 3: SITUATIONAL BEHAVIOR

Review

Review the "Therapist Rules for Administering Step 3" in the text (pp. 123–125) and summarized here:

1. Provide a rationale to the patient for Step 3 (text, pp. 123–124).
2. Teach the patient to monitor his/her situational behavior and to keep track of those behaviors that lead to the achievement of desired outcomes.

Review the "Patient Performance Goal for Step 3" in the text, p. 125) and summarized here:

1. Patient learns to focus on relevant aspects of his/her behavior that lead to the achievement of the desired outcome.

Sample Criterion Behavioral Pinpointing

"On Tuesday my office mate listened to a rock station on his radio all day—from 8 A.M. to 5 P.M. He does this several times a week. I can't get any work done because I cannot concentrate. I wanted him to turn off the radio. I should have told him what I wanted, but I didn't say anything. I just kept quiet and got mad. I stayed angry all day and just thought about how inconsiderate he was. Tuesday ended, and I went home really mad and depressed."

Behavioral problem(s): Lack of assertive behavior requesting that the radio be turned off or down, or wearing earplugs.

Exercises

Following are 10 situational behavior exercises. For each:

1. Read the scenarios and pinpoint the behavioral problem(s) that need work.
2. After completing each exercise, *check your responses with the criterion answers on pp. 81–83.*

Note. It is important to remember that actual skill training and rehearsal for behavioral problems are not undertaken during the SA. However, SA accomplishes two behavioral goals: (1) Therapists (privately) pinpoint the patient's behavioral problems during Step 3 of the elicitation phase; and (2) they help the patient target the behaviors needed to obtain the desired outcome during Step 2 of the remediation phase. You will complete the first behavioral task in the exercises below.

Situational Behavior 1

"I gave the cashier a $20 bill for a 55¢ purchase. The cashier told me that I had to take 19 singles for my change. *I saw that she had a drawer full of tens and fives.* I just stood there and watched her count out 19 singles and some change. I didn't want all of those singles, but I just held out my hand and she gave them to me."

a. Behavioral problem(s):

_____

_____

_____

_____

b. *Did your behavioral target(s) agree with the criterion answer on p. 81? If not, what were the differences?* _____

Situational Behavior 2

"My husband told me that the dinner I cooked was terrible. He called me a bad cook. He went on and on with his criticism. I just listened to his ranting and raving without saying anything. Just sat there and picked at my food. I feel like a total failure."

a. Behavioral problem(s):

_____

_____

_____

_____

b. *Did your behavioral target(s) agree with the criterion answer on p. 81? If not, what were the differences?* _____

Situational Behavior 3

"I told my employee off. He made a stupid mistake adding up a sales bill total with a customer. He tried to explain what had gone wrong and why he'd made the mistake. I just got madder and told him that if he makes another mistake like this again, I'll fire him. He's my best salesman, but I really lost it, and I laid into him."

a. Behavioral problem(s):

_____

_____

_____

_____

b. *Did your behavioral target(s) agree with the criterion answer on p. 81? If not, what were the differences?* _____

Situational Behavior 4

"I asked my husband to help me with the housework, and he became angry with me. He told me he wouldn't help me do anything! He said that I ought to see that he was watching TV. I didn't say anything else to him. He always reacts that way when I ask for his help. That night he came to bed, all sweet, and wanted to have sex as if nothing had happened. After we did it, he fell right off to sleep. It took me a long time to go to sleep. I was still feeling hurt."

a. Behavioral problem(s):

_____

_____

_____

_____

b. *Did your behavioral target(s) agree with the criterion answer on p. 81? If not, what were the differences?* _____

Situational Behavior 5

"I had a wonderful evening and really enjoyed the time we spent together. She seemed to feel the same way. I just didn't know how to take things further. I didn't say anything to her at the door to her apartment, when she kissed me and asked me to come in. Just stood there wondering what to do. The next thing I said was that I had had a really nice time. Then I turned around and walked to my car and drove off. I felt like a fool!"

a. Behavioral problem(s):

_____

_____

_____

_____

b. *Did your behavioral target(s) agree with the criterion answer on pp. 81–82? If not, what were the differences?* _____

Situational Behavior 6

"Last Saturday evening, my boyfriend and I got into a big argument about what we wanted to do. I wanted to go out to eat first, and he wanted to go to a movie and then go out to eat. I did something that I have never done before. I told him that I always become frustrated and angry when people don't do what I want. I also said that I am trying to change and do things differently. Then I said, 'Look, let's go the movie, and then we can get something to eat.' Things really worked out well, and the evening was great fun. He asked me to go out next weekend and said we must go to eat before we do anything else."

a. Behavioral problem(s):

_____

_____

_____

_____

b. *Did your behavioral target(s) agree with the criterion answer on p. 82? If not, what were the differences?* _____

Situational Behavior 7

Note: This patient (male) has made only fleeting eye contact with the therapist (female). Whenever he talks, he looks to the left, to the right, or down at the floor.

"My date told me last night that I needed to be more assertive. She said that I never look at her. I don't know where that came from. We had been having dinner at a restaurant, and I thought the evening was going okay. I didn't reply to her. I just shrugged my shoulders, and told her that I thought I was assertive enough."

a. Behavioral problem(s):

_____

_____

_____

_____

b. *Did your behavioral target(s) agree with the criterion answer on p. 82? If not, what were the differences?* _____

Situational Behavior 8

Note: This patient laughs frequently whenever she talks about herself. This pattern is particularly noticeable whenever she wants something or actually asks for something.

"I went to the cleaners Monday to take my blouses to be laundered. I wanted to pick them up the next day. The clerk told me this would be impossible [patient said that she laughed while talking to the clerk]. I told her that I needed them right away [patient noted that she smiled at the clerk and laughed again]. The clerk became a little more upset [patient reported laughing once more] and told me they would be ready Wednesday evening at the earliest. [Patient said she started to get angry but laughed once more and said to the clerk that the cleaners advertise 'next day service.' The clerk retorted that it was 'Wednesday or nothing' and the patient said she laughed again.] I gathered up my blouses and told her, 'Forget it!' [again, she laughed when she said this to the clerk]. I left the store."

a. Behavioral problem(s):

_____

_____

_____

_____

b. *Did your behavioral target(s) agree with the criterion answer on p. 82? If not, what were the differences?* _____

Situational Behavior 9

"I am a member of our church committee that is studying our space needs on Sunday morning to determine if we need to enlarge the sanctuary. We only had a few members show up for the last meeting. I should have called everyone to remind them about the meeting. I told the group that I should have called everyone and that the poor attendance was my fault. The people who were there tried to tell me that it was not my job to call everyone and remind them. I just kept saying that 'it was my fault.' I felt responsible. We went round and round about this for a long time. I kept saying the same thing, even though they disagreed with me. They never did convince me otherwise. We never got anything done at the meeting."

a. Behavioral problem(s):

_____

_____

_____

_____

b. *Did your behavioral target(s) agree with the criterion answer on pp. 82–83? If not, what were the differences?* _____

Situational Behavior 10

"I told my 10-year-old child that she could not wear her dress so short. She starting arguing with me. In fact, she really got mad at me. I tried to stand my ground and give her all the reasons why I thought her dress was too short, and why I thought it would be socially inappropriate for her to wear it this way. Finally, I told her: 'Just forget about it; it's not that important anyway. Just do what you want to do and wear your short skirt to school.' When she went to school, I was furious with myself for being such a wimp."

a. Behavioral problem(s):

_____

_____

_____

_____

b. *Did your behavioral target(s) agree with the criterion answer on p. 83? If not, what were the differences?* _____

Criterion Answers for Step 3 Elicitation Exercises

Situational Behavior 1

Problem: Lack of assertive behavior accompanied by a goal-directed focus.

Solution: The patient must decide on a desired outcome (DO) that would focus his/her behavior in an effective direction. For example, would he/she ask for larger bills, since they were visible in the register drawer? Would he/she say that if the change had to be made in singles, then he/she would shop elsewhere?

Situational Behavior 2

Problem: Lack of assertive behavior with the husband.

Solution: The initial behavioral response should be directed toward giving feedback to the husband concerning the effects of his hurtful comments on the patient. A choice point then arises for the patient: Does the patient want to pursue (1) why her husband wants to hurt her in this manner or (2) the issue of what the husband wants to do about the obvious "food problem."

Situational Behavior 3

Problem: Lack of anger control; lack of goal-directed behavior regarding employee problems.

Solution: A focus on helping the patient learn to teach adaptable behavior to his employees rather than punishing misbehavior (i.e., making mistakes when totaling the sales bill) is the best way to teach anger control in this instance. This is an old operant tactic that frequently works. I would also tell the patient that controlling his anger in such situations takes pre-planning: I would ask him to list anticipated problem situations with employees and we would work out similar teaching strategies.

Situational Behavior 4

Problem: Lack of assertive feedback behavior with the husband.

Solution: Patient must learn to provide immediate feedback to the husband whenever he hurts her with comments such as this. The husband is also unaware that his request for sex is incongruent following such injurious exchanges and that having sex at such a time poses notable interpersonal difficulties for the patient. The husband is clearly not aware of the negative consequences his behavior is having on his wife.

Situational Behavior 5

Problem: Lack of assertive behavior accompanied by goal-directed focus; social skills deficit around females (inconclusive).

Solution: Patient must learn to pinpoint what he wants to do in the situation (this involves the DO), and then let the other person know. It may be that once the patient is able to tell the woman what he wants in an appropriate manner, no further social skills training will be necessary. If glaring social inadequacies with females are present, then formal training will have to be instituted.

Situational Behavior 6

Problem: None present; the patient behaved appropriately.

Situational Behavior 7

Problem: Inappropriate interpersonal behavior (inability to make eye contact with the therapist and others).

Solution: The therapist must teach the patient to maintain appropriate eye contact with him/her first. Then the skill must be transferred outside of therapy. Constant feedback from the clinician should be administered for this behavior, particularly when good eye contact is being maintained.

Situational Behavior 8

Problem: Incongruence between the patient's verbal and nonverbal behavior channels.

Solution: Laughter that is emitted when a person is trying to be serious sends confusing messages. Laughter is a nonverbal signal that communicates the following: "This is a light exchange and do not take me seriously." The verbal content of the patient's presentation to the clerk was very serious. Laughing while being serious sends a conflicting and confusing message—the laughter cancels out the serious content, and vice versa. This patient will have to learn to make serious declarative sentences without smiling or laughing. This behavior skill training can be accomplished during the therapy hour after the SA is completed. It is not unusual for such patients to have difficulty taking themselves seriously when they want something. This component may be motivating the nonverbal laughter during serious encounters.

Situational Behavior 9

Problem: Inability to take seriously what others say and then behave accordingly.

Solution: This patient's DO was to help the group have a productive meeting. The meeting was nonproductive and the DO was not obtained because the patient could not take seriously what the group was trying to say to her. It is not unusual for these patients to have difficulty taking what the therapist says seriously, particularly when it involves some aspect of their behavior. The place to begin training is during the exchanges between the patient and the therapist. Exposing the fact that the patient finds it difficult to believe the therapist and questioning why this might be the case will evoke the necessary historical problems that must be addressed to remedy the problem.

Situational Behavior 10

Problem: Being unable to maintain effective behavioral limits on a 10-year-old child.

Solution: As in the above exercises, this patient may find it difficult to take seriously her own decisions concerning child-raising. If this is the case, the question becomes *why*. Assisting the patient to attribute greater credibility to her own limit-setting and supporting/reinforcing such behavior is clearly indicated. It will never be easy or stress-free—certainly not with children or adolescents!

STEP 4: ACTUAL OUTCOME

Review

Review the "Therapist Rules for Administering Step 4" in the text (pp. 125–129) and summarized here:

1. Provide a rationale to the patient for Step 4 (text, pp. 125–126).
2. Frame the AO in a time-anchored sentence that is constructed in behavioral terms (stated so that an observer could see it happen).
3. Do not construct AOs in emotional terms.
4. Do not paraphrase or alter the patient's AO construction.
5. Let the patient do the work of AO construction.

Review the "Patient Performance Goal for Step 4" in the text (p. 129) and summarized here:

1. The patient learns to construct the AO in one sentence using behavioral terminology.

Exercises

1. Construct an AO sentence for each situational description. Remember, the AO denotes the exit/endpoint of the situation. *If* the situational description is presented in such a way that AO construction becomes difficult/impossible to determine, then diagnose the problem in the space provided.
2. After completing each exercise, *check your responses with the criterion answers on pp. 89–91.*

Actual Outcome 1

"I talked to my neighbor this morning about his bass boat being parked on the edge of my property. I asked him to move the boat so that it would be off my property line. Finally, he said, 'Okay, I'll move the boat to the other side of the yard.' He moved his boat."

Write out the AO sentence or diagnose the problem:

_____

_____

How did your AO response compare with the criterion answer on p. 89? _____

_____

Actual Outcome 2

"I called the hostess of our convention to tell her how I wanted the room set up. She and I started talking, and I described how I wanted the room arranged. I explained my thoughts about how the chairs should be positioned. The more I talked with her the more anxious I became. She said that my arrangement ideas were good and that she would implement them. When the conversation ended, I was so nervous thinking about my ideas being implemented that I could barely focus on what she had said to me."

Write out the AO sentence or diagnose the problem:

_____

_____

How did your AO response compare with the criterion answer on p. 89? _____

_____

Actual Outcome 3

"Our big project was due on Friday and my colleagues and I talked in the conference room one last time. Jane listed the unfinished steps that involved her staff. Bill did the same for his staff. When it was my turn to review the progress of my staff, I presented two things. After I finished, the group said they were pleased with my overall work. The meeting broke up, and I continued to talk to Fred, whose staff had completed his part of the project. He told me about his son and how his family had gone to his hockey game on Monday night. His son was obviously the star of the team. We agreed to meet later and talk about the hockey game over a beer."

Write out the AO sentence or diagnose the problem:

_____

_____

How did your AO response compare with the criterion answer on p. 89? _____

_____

Actual Outcome 4

"I called Mary and asked her to go to the opera with me on Saturday evening. She said that she would. I was so excited that I almost dropped the phone. I worked out the time I would pick her up. Then I called my buddy and told him the good news. We talked about the conversation I had just had with Mary, and he told me that I was one lucky guy!"

Write out the AO sentence or diagnose the problem:

_____

_____

How did your AO response compare with the criterion answer on p. 89? _____

_____

Actual Outcome 5

"My plant colleague and I have been working on plans for a new wing design for a new Lockeed airplane. We had frequent arguments during our conversation on Monday morning. On Tuesday we seemed to agree more on the aerodynamic specifications, but we ended the day at each other's throats again—arguing and in total disagreement. Wednesday, we didn't talk much. Friday was another conflictual day. He and I started arguing in the morning, and it went on all day. By 5 P.M. on Friday I was exhausted, so I left the office without telling Bill good-bye."

Write out the AO sentence or diagnose the problem:

_____

_____

How did your AO response compare with the criterion answer on p. 90? _____

_____

Actual Outcome 6

"For the past week my wife and I have been talking about remodeling our living room and den. We have gone over every inch of both rooms, discussing and debating what we want and don't want. It seemed at times that our disagreements were not resolvable. The final issue was where to put the entertainment center in the den. She wanted it near the fireplace on the north wall, and I wanted it across the room on the south wall. We compromised by deciding to put the fireplace in the middle of the den with a wrap-around see-through fire screen. The discussion was finished, and we agreed on everything."

Write out the AO sentence or diagnose the problem:

_____

_____

How did your AO response compare with the criterion answer on p. 90? _____

_____

Actual Outcome 7

"I always get so flustered whenever I have to defend my opinion on something. This is especially true when what I say conflicts with someone else's opinion. I wish I could stand my ground, feel confident, and talk in a reasonable way. Earlier this week, I got into another one of those situations. My cousin from Seattle was visiting me, and she said she wanted to go see the movie *The Man on the Moon*. I told her, 'I hate Andy Kaufman and this movie is the last one I want to see.' The *American President* was also on, and I said I wanted to go see this one. We got into a debate over which movie would be better. Once again, I became flustered and had no confidence in my position."

Write out the AO sentence or diagnose the problem:

_____

_____

How did your AO response compare with the criterion answer on p. 90? _____

_____

Actual Outcome 8

"I was audited by the I.R.S. this week. The agent came to the house in the evening, and my husband and I sat around the kitchen table and pulled out all our records and receipts for 1998. He went through the tax return we had filed (line by line) and made some adjustments. However, two or three major adjustments had to be made because we had added our 1998 gross income totals incorrectly. It meant that we still owed a considerable amount of money on the 1998 return. We all agreed on what the refund total was, and the agent thanked us for our time and left."

Write out the AO sentence or diagnose the problem:

_____

_____

How did your AO response compare with the criterion answer on p. 90? _____

_____

Actual Outcome 9

"I finally asserted myself to my supervisor. He was pointing out all the mistakes I had made in my last report. It had been a hurry-up job request because he had to present our department's sales data to the CEO and board. Instead of getting mad and pouting, like I usually do when this happens, I reacted to his comments differently this time. I told him that I did the best I could, given the severe time constraints. He acknowledged that I didn't have enough time to do a thorough job."

Write out the AO sentence or diagnose the problem:

_____

_____

How did your AO response compare with the criterion answer on p. 90? _____

_____

Actual Outcome 10

"My girlfriend and I had another argument last night. We just don't know how to settle arguments once they arise. She wanted to go out to eat, and I wanted to stay home and cook steaks. Doesn't sound like that big a deal when I tell it, but by the time the argument ended, it had become a major crisis. We called each other bad names and insinuated all sorts of negative things about one another. The argument was never resolved and I went home mad."

Write out the AO sentence or diagnose the problem:

_____

_____

How did your AO response compare with the criterion answer on p. 91? _____

_____

Criterion Answers for Step 4 Elicitation Exercises

Actual Outcome 1

Problem: Resolved.

Note: The sentence "He moved his boat," denotes the exit/endpoint of the situation. It is stated in behavioral terms so that an observer can see it. Patients must learn to construct their AOs in a similar manner. The clearer the exit point, the easier it is to show patients the consequences of their behavior.

Actual Outcome 2

Problem: The patient must learn to frame the AO in behavioral terms. The correct AO would be the following: "The hostess said that my arrangement ideas were good and she agreed to implement them." It is acceptable for patients to describe how they felt emotionally at the end of the situation, as long as they construct the AO in behavioral terms.

Note: If you have further questions about why we avoid using emotional language in the AO and work only with behaviorally framed AOs (see p. 127 in the text).

Actual Outcome 3

Problem: Phillip has included another situational event at the end of the first one that involved the meeting in the conference room. The therapist must insist that the patient stay with one situation and state an AO for that situation: "The group said they were pleased with my overall work."

Note: Chronically depressed patients often shift their focus from one topic to another. Therapists must teach patients to concentrate on only one slice-of-time in SA. Otherwise, the behavioral consequences (AO) in the situation will be lost in an avalanche of extraneous information.

Actual Outcome 4

Problem: The patient has again shifted from one situation to a second event that followed on the heels of his conversation with Mary. The correct AO would be: "Mary accepted my offer of a date, and we worked out the time."

Note: One reason it is important to remain focused on the encounter with Mary is because the patient's behavior has led to success with Mary. If the clinician allows the patient to insert the scenario with the buddy, the patient's success consequences may get lost in the tangent. Taking the opportunity to highlight the patient's successful behavior with Mary is the effective strategy.

Actual Outcome 5

Problem: We cannot determine an AO because several situations are included in the situational description. The correct therapeutic maneuver here is to ask the patient to select *one day* out of the week and describe his argumentative encounter with Bill. Based on the information we have, it really doesn't matter which day is selected—just have the individual select one.

Actual Outcome 6

Problem: Resolved.

Note: Notice how circuitous the interactional path was from the beginning to the exit/ endpoint, "My wife and I agreed on how to remodel our whole house." This is fine and often reflective of how interactions proceed between mature individuals. Relevant and accurate interpretations help patients remain grounded during these interactive twists and turns. If patients are anchored when they face a serious disagreement, their own relevant and accurate interpretations frequently enable them to resolve the disagreement by the time the exit point of the situation is reached.

Actual Outcome 7

Problem: The situational description has *no* exit/endpoint; therefore we cannot determine an AO. We don't know if the debate between the patient and the cousin is the outcome, if they ever went to a movie, or if there is another outcome. The therapist must help the person determine the exit/endpoint of the situation, and then construct an AO.

Note: Remember to avoid the error of leaving the AO in emotional terms (e.g., "flustered and had no confidence," etc.), even though this is the last comment the patient made in the situational description.

Actual Outcome 8

Problem: Resolved.

Note: The AO formulation, "The refund total was agreed upon," is clearly presented in the situational description.

Actual Outcome 9

Problem: Resolved.

Note: The AO, "My supervisor acknowledged that I had insufficient time to prepare a mistake-free report," is clearly presented in the situational description.

Actual Outcome 10

Problem: Unresolved argument, but outcome correctly stated at the endpoint of the situation.

Note: The AO, "The argument was never resolved and I went home mad," is formulated in behavioral terms. Again, it is acceptable for patients to describe the way they felt when they exited the situation, as long as the AO is stated in behavioral terms.

STEP 5: DESIRED OUTCOME

Review

Review the "Therapist Rules for Administering Step 5" in the text (pp. 131–138) and summarized here:

1. Provide a rationale to the patient for Step 5 (text, p. 131).
2. Teach patient to construct only one behaviorally defined DO per SA.
3. Teach patient to construct *attainable* (the environment can/will deliver/produce the DO) and *realistic* (the patient has the capacity to produce the outcome) DOs.
4. Be sure you understand every word in the DO sentence.
5. Let the patient do the work of constructing the DO.
6. If the DO is achieved, *but* there is verbal/nonverbal distress evident in the patient (or the therapist) concerning the DO, the DO must be revised.

Review the "Patient Performance Goals for Step 5" in the text (p. 138) and summarized here:

1. Patient learns to construct one behaviorally defined DO per SA.
2. Patient learns to construct *attainable* and *realistic* DOs.

Exercises

Following are 10 DO exercises. For each:

1. Read each situation and formulate the DO for it and/or answer the questions about the DO.
2. In situations where patients have left the DO in the hands of the environment (an attainable versus unattainable issue), decide if the DO is attainable (use the *attainability* criteria in the text, pp. 133–134).
3. After each exercise, *check your work with the criterion answers on pp. 98–100.*

Desired Outcome 1

"I wanted Jim to take the lead at our next meeting and chair the proceedings. I have been the chair for the last three sessions. Jim and I talked about my role as chair, and I repeatedly said I was tired of doing it. I kept hoping he would volunteer to be the chair. We reviewed the entire agenda for the coming meeting, and we went over each item one by one. Jim never once volunteered to chair the meeting. Finally, we stopped talking about the meeting and went back to our offices."

Patient's situational DO: "I wanted Jim to volunteer to chair the proceedings at our next meeting."

a. Given the situational description, is the DO attainable? (Yes/No) Why?

_____

_____

_____

b. What must be *added to* the situation to help the patient determine if the DO is attainable? (See text, pp. 152–153.)

_____

_____

Check your answers with the criterion answers on p. 98.

Desired Outcome 2

"I talked to my dad and asked him to call us before he comes over to visit Betty and me. He agreed to try to remember to do this but asked why this was necessary. 'After all, you're my son,' he said. I explained that sometimes it might not be convenient for us to have visitors and that Betty might have other plans, not be dressed, or just not want visitors at that time. He said he understood what I was saying, and he agreed to call the next time."

a. Given the situational description, construct the DO for this situation:

_____

_____

b. Does your DO meet the attainable/realistic criteria? (See text, pp. 133–135.) (Yes/No)
c. Explain why for each:

_____

_____

Check your answers with the criterion answers on p. 98.

Desired Outcome 3

"I'm coaching a T-Ball Little League team, and I wanted the team members to bag up all the equipment and put the bag in my car before they left practice. Today, we had a team meeting before practice started. I reminded all the team members that I wanted them to help bag up all the equipment before they left the field to meet their parents. I asked them if they would comply with my request and the group unanimously said, 'Yes.' When the last kid was picked up, all the equipment had been bagged. The bag had been put in the trunk of my car. I was delighted."

a. Construct a realistic DO for the situation:

_____

_____

b. Construct an attainable DO for the situation:

_____

_____

Check your answers with the criterion answers on p. 98.

Desired Outcome 4

"The mission committee at our church met last Wednesday night. The major issue was where would we send our mission monies this year. There were 20 people present, and everyone had an opinion. My own feeling was that the monies ought to go to a place where the need was the greatest. I presented my decision-making rationale to the group. My hope was that the group would use this rationale to make the choice. After hearing the list of needy sites, I proposed that my selection rationale be used for making the decision. The group felt this was the best way to make the choice. Someone then nominated a small group of churches in Appalachia as the site with the greatest need. The money will go to the Appalachian churches."

a. Based on the situational description, construct a realistic DO for the situation:

_____

_____

Check your answers with the criterion answers on p. 98.

Desired Outcome 5

"My next-door neighbor and I discussed how to combine our outdoor Christmas tree lights so that both yards would look good and be color coordinated. Both yards have a lot of trees, and our property lines are right next to each other with no fence in between. We discussed using our white lights for the trees, and he wanted to place the red and green lights in the bushes and shrubs. This sounded okay to me. We still had some light strings left, particularly some long strings of blue lights. I wanted him to suggest that we run the strings of blue lights across the front of both houses. We ended the discussion, and he never did volunteer to do what I wanted. The blue light strings and what to do with them were never discussed."

Patient's situational DO: "I wanted Phil to suggest that we use the blue light strings to run across the front of both houses."

a. What attainability problem is present in the DO?

_____

_____

b. What must be *added to* the situation to help the patient determine if the DO is attainable?

_____

_____

c. Based on the situational description, we don't know if the DO is attainable or not, so write out a realistic DO for the situation:

_____

_____

Check your answers with the criterion answers on pp. 98–99.

Desired Outcome 6

"I've never been able to stand up to my husband when we disagree. It happened again this past Sunday morning. He didn't like the scrambled eggs I fixed, and he said: 'You are the worst cook I've ever known! These eggs are terrible!' He hurt my feelings by his comments. I told him that I'd tried to cook them the way he liked. He never answered me. I left the room, went into the bedroom, and cried for 30 minutes."

Patient's situational DO: "I wish my husband wouldn't treat me this way."

a. Is the DO attainable? (Yes/No)
b. Write out a realistic DO for the situation:

_____

_____

c. What must be *added to* the situation before the patient can construct a realistic DO?

_____

_____

Check your answers with the criterion answers on p. 99.

Desired Outcome 7

"I'm the team quarterback and we were on the opponents' 7-yard-line with 10 seconds left in the game. I called a timeout and went over to talk with the coach. I told my coach that the right side of the line had been moving the defensive lineman out every time we ran Trap 39. Our pulling tackle had also taken out the left outside linebacker each time we ran the play. I wanted to call this same play again and try to score. He thought about my plan for a few seconds, then told me to call Trap 39. I did, and we won the game on the final play."

a. Write out a realistic DO for the situation:

_____

_____

Check your answer with the criterion answers on p. 99.

Desired Outcome 8

"I went to see my graduate economics teaching assistant to ask if I could take my final exam a few days late. I told her that my sister was having a serious spinal cord operation on the day of the exam. She lived in another city, and if I went, I would have to drive several hours to get there. I would need to leave the day before the exam, because the surgery was scheduled for 7:30 A.M. on exam day. I would not be coming back to the university until Friday of exam week. I laid out the reasons as clearly as I could. I asked her if I could take the exam late. She told me that she didn't have the authority to give me permission to take the exam late—that I would have to speak directly to the professor."

Patient's situational DO: "I wanted the TA to give me permission to take the exam late."

a. Based on the situational description, is the DO attainable? (Yes/No)
b. How would the DO have to be revised to make it realistic?

_____

_____

Check your answers with the criterion answers on p. 99.

Desired Outcome 9

"I have a severe rotator cuff problem in my right shoulder that has messed up my pitching career. I haven't been able to pitch for 6 months. I went to see my orthopedic doctor last Wednesday, and he examined the injury after X-raying the shoulder. He told me that I needed surgery and that it would be a year before I would know whether I could pitch again. I left his office feeling depressed and discouraged.

Patient's situational DO: "I wanted my shoulder to be well by now."

a. Are there problems with this patient's DO? (Yes/No)
b. Is the DO an *unattainable* or *unrealistic* one? Explain why.

_____

_____

c. Construct a realistic DO for the situation:

_____

_____

Check your answers with the criterion answers on p. 99.

Desired Outcome 10

"I have worked through all the above DO exercises. I think I understand how to construct DOs using the attainable and realistic criteria. However, I still find that I have to stop and think before I make a decision about the adequacy of a DO."

CBASP Trainee's DO: "I want to get where I can make this assessment automatically (with little or no thought)."

a. Is the DO realistic? (Yes/No)
b. What might be a more realistic DO for you? Write out a revised DO:

_____

_____

Check your answers with the criterion answers on pp. 99–100.

Criterion Answers for Step 5 Elicitation Exercises

Desired Outcome 1

a. No, not under the present circumstances. The patient never asked Jim specifically to take over as chair. Persuasion by "indirect suggestions" is always a risky strategy. It is clear that Jim (the environment) will not voluntarily take over the chair role.

b. An action read, such as "I've got to ask Jim if he will be chair," must be inserted to prompt assertive behavior and make the DO explicit. Then, and only then, will the patient know if his DO is attainable. (See text, pp. 152–153.)

Desired Outcome 2

a. "Dad will agree to call us before he comes over to our house."

b. Yes.

c. The DO is attainable because the father (the environment) agreed to comply with the request to call before coming to visit. The DO could also be formulated in realistic terms: "I *want to ask* my Dad to call before coming to visit." As it stands now, obtaining a verbal agreement from the father places the DO in the hands of the environment, but in this case, it is attainable.

Desired Outcome 3

a. "Before leaving practice, I want to ask the team members to bag up the equipment and put the bag in my car."

b. "I want the entire team to agree to bag up the equipment and put the bag in my car before leaving."

Desired Outcome 4

a. "I wanted to propose to the mission committee that we give our monies to the site with the greatest need."

Desired Outcome 5

a. The patient never told his neighbor what he wanted to do with the blue light strings. This is a common occurrence. Chronic patients want others to know what they want without having to ask or having to make their desires known. Since the neighbor didn't know how the patient wanted to use the blue lights, the DO was not achieved.

b. An action interpretation such as, "I've got to ask Phil to string the blue lights across the front of his house," followed by a specific request, may have made the DO obtainable. Had Phil said, "No," then the DO would remain unattainable.

c. "I want to ask Phil to string his blue lights across the front of his house."

Note: Realistic DOs are always safer goals and easier to achieve. Attainable DOs leave the locus of control in another person's court and are always riskier. However, attainable DOs always define what the environment will and will not deliver, once the patient makes explicit what he/she wants.

Desired Outcome 6

a. No. The husband *does* treat her this way and the wishful thinking that characterizes this DO will not modify the husband's behavior.
b. "I must tell my husband how much his comment just hurt my feelings."
c. An action read to prompt an assertive reply to the husband.

Note: Sometimes this type of feedback to spouses has a salutary effect. I have seen cases where blatant rudeness and insensitive behavior like the kind described in this scenario were modified when patients began to provide direct feedback to the spouse.

Desired Outcome 7

a. "I want to tell my coach why I want to run Trap 39 on the final play of the game."

Desired Outcome 8

a. No. The situational event makes the DO unattainable (the environment represented by the TA cannot produce the DO). Unfortunately, this is not an unusual DO among chronically depressed adults. They often want what is not attainable.
b. "I want to ask the TA to let me take the exam late."

Desired Outcome 9

a. Yes.
b. Yes. It is an unrealistic DO. Wishful thinking, a common coping strategy for chronic patients, is the basis for this DO. The patient cannot produce a "well" shoulder at the present time.
c. "I want a current diagnosis on the state of my shoulder" or "I want to get a second medical opinion."

Note: These are realistic DOs that are achievable and that focus the patient's energy on the problem at hand.

Desired Outcome 10

a. No. The DO is unrealistic (no one can make DO assessments automatically—it takes careful thought).
b. "I want to improve my DO decision-making skills by continual practice."

Note: No CBASP therapist ever reaches the place where DO adequacy decisions are easy. This is because patients keep bringing us new variations of DOs that we haven't encountered. Keep working at it. Your performance will improve over time. Teaching patients to live within the bounds of realistic and attainable DOs always remains a laborious task. I have known CBASP therapists (and I must include myself) who don't always live within these boundaries!

STEP 6: COMPARING THE AO AND THE DO

Review

Review the "Therapist Rules for Administering Step 6" in the text (pp. 139–140) and summarized here:

1. State the AO versus DO question clearly and do not rush the patient through Step 6 (text, pp. 139–140).
2. Ask the patient *why* he/she did/did not achieve the DO *only after* allowing sufficient time for the patient to make the AO versus DO comparison.

Review the "Patient Performance Goal for Step 6" in the text (pp. 140–141) and summarized here:

1. Patient learns to evaluate the efficacy of his/her situational behavior using the AO versus DO comparison.

Exercises

Following are four AO/DO comparisons. For each:

1. Read each verbatim scenario and evaluate the therapist's Step 6 behavior.
2. Check your answers with the criterion answers on p. 104.

AO/DO Comparison 1

THERAPIST: You got what you wanted in this situation, didn't you?

PATIENT: Yes.

THERAPIST: You got it because you told your partner exactly what you wanted. Isn't this why you achieved the DO here?

PATIENT: Yes.

a. Write out your evaluation of the therapist's behavior in light of the Step 6 criteria: ____
_____
_____

b. What would you do to remedy any problems you mentioned above? Be specific. _____
_____
_____

Check your answers with the criterion answers on p. 104.

AO/DO Comparison 2

THERAPIST: Your DO was that you wanted to tell your wife that she hurt you when she answered your questions so abruptly. Your AO stated that you did just this. Did you get what you wanted in the situation?

PATIENT: Yes, I finally did it! I finally told her what effect she had on me.

THERAPIST: Why do you think you got what you wanted?

PATIENT: Because I finally asserted myself. She listened to me and apologized for hurting me. God, it has taken me long enough to do this, hasn't it?

a. Write out your evaluation of the therapist's performance in light of the Step 6 criteria: _
   _____
   _____

b. Do you see any problems? If so, what are they? _____
   _____

Check your answers with the criterion answers on p. 104.

AO/DO Comparison 3

THERAPIST: Did you get what you wanted in the situation?

PATIENT: Yes, I did. I prepared well and knew exactly what I was going to say.

THERAPIST: The reason you achieved your DO here was because you had prepared well for the presentation. You have convinced me that you have difficulty organizing your thoughts when you speak extemporaneously. I have also thought that many of your problems arise because you don't think first, you just react. Some people call it impulsive behavior. I'm not going to get into all that labeling of your behavior, but thinking it through, what you wanted to do before you acted surely seemed to make a difference here. I hope you have learned this lesson well. I think it will serve you well in the future.

PATIENT: You're right.

a. Write out your evaluation of the therapist's performance in light of the Step 6 criteria: _
   _____
   _____

b. Would you have administered this task any differently? If so, write out what you would have done: _____
   _____
   _____

Check your answers with the criterion answers on p. 104.

AO/DO Comparison 4

THERAPIST: Did you get what you wanted in this situation?

PATIENT: Yes.

THERAPIST: (*after an appropriate pause*) Why do you think you obtained your DO?

PATIENT: Because I prepared my remarks ahead of time. I don't do well when I have to speak extemporaneously.

a. Write out your evaluation of the therapist's performance in light of the Step 6 criteria:

_____

_____

b. Would you have done anything differently? If so, write out what you would have done:

_____

_____

Check your answers with the criterion answers on p. 104.

Criterion Answers for Step 6 Elicitation Exercises

AO/DO Comparison 1

a. Unacceptable performance. The AO versus DO question was never asked, nor the "why" question. Instead, the clinician did the work for the patient by telling him/her why the DO was obtained.

b. Ask two questions here:
   1. "Did you get what you wanted here?" Wait for a complete answer, then ask:
   2. "Why did you get what you wanted?" Wait for a complete answer.

AO/DO Comparison 2

a. Excellent therapist performance; adheres to all of Step 6 criteria.

b. No. Prompt questions are acceptable, and the patient does the work.

AO/DO Comparison 3

a. Unacceptable performance. Therapist begins the step correctly by asking the AO versus DO question. Then, instead of asking the "why" question, the clinician begins preaching to the patient, telling him why the DO was achieved. This is a common error among new CBASP therapists. Waiting for the patient to do the work of therapy is difficult. It is so much easier to do the work yourself. It is also a lethal tactic and one that you and I must learn to inhibit.

b. Yes! I would have asked the "why" question and then let the patient provide the reason(s) why the DO was achieved.

AO/DO Comparison 4

a. Excellent performance. The therapist asks the correct Step 6 questions, and the patient does all the work.

b. No. Excellent work.

PART II
Situational Analysis: Remediation Phase Exercises

During the remediation phase, patients "fix" badly managed interpersonal situations wherein they failed to obtain the desired outcome (i.e., where the AO ≠ DO). Repairing situations by correcting the cognitive and behavioral errors that precluded attainment of the DO is the goal of remediation. Patients first confront the negative consequences of their behavior during the elicitation phase of SA. Then they work to avoid repeating the mistakes that resulted in negative consequences by revising old behaviors and replacing them with new ones. Remediation of a badly managed interpersonal encounter achieves four objectives:

- It demonstrates that behavior has predictable consequences.
- It accentuates the truism that unless patients change their behavior, failure and misery will continue.
- It targets the specific cognitions and behaviors that must be modified if the DO is to be achieved.
- It transfers in-session SA learning to the everyday living arena.

During the early sessions, after fixing the original situation and inserting adaptable cognitive and behavioral strategies that would lead to the attainment of the DO, patients sometimes remark: "I could never do this outside the therapy session." The most effective strategy is to assure patients that they don't have to. The next therapist comment is important because it highlights the negative reinforcement ramifications that must be understood in order to prompt and motivate the new behavior.

> "You and I will continue to talk about strategies that will get you what you want, and we will do this in the safety of the session. That's what SA is all about. When you get tired of producing the old consequences and when you're ready to achieve your desired outcome, then at least you'll know what you have to do and how you will have to do it. It's up to you."

Cognitive dissonance is created by this comment, particularly when the SA has addressed problems the patient is having with a valued interpersonal partner. Implicated are two contradictory pieces of information: (1) desirable conditions are within the patient's grasp (even though fear-engendering to reach for) because he/she knows how to produce them; (2) the safety of the passive status quo behaviors are now associated with a fear-avoidance motif and have acquired negative connotations. More often than not, these patients will come to the next session reporting that they have reduced the dissonance between the desired new condition and the safety of the old way by doing what they said they could not do. They also frequently report (with much relief) that they achieved the DO. Success events such as these also increase the patient's motivation to change.

The remediation phase includes four steps. *Step 1* revises those interpretations constructed during the elicitation phase that are irrelevant and/or inaccurate. The completion of Step 1 frequently requires that faulty cognitive interpretations be revised if the DO is to be obtained.

In *Step 2* inappropriate behavior is replaced with more effective maneuvers. In *Step 3* the new learning is summarized, and *Step 4* transfers and generalizes SA learning to relationship situations on the outside. When the remediation phase is finished, patients have taken a problematical situation wherein the DO was not obtained, identified the cognitive and behavioral problems that precluded DO attainment, revised the ineffective strategies, summarized the relevant learning, and transferred the new learning to other interpersonal relationships.

STEP 1: REMEDIATION OF THE INTERPRETATIONS

Review

See "Therapist Rules for Administering Step 1" in the text (pp. 148–157) and summarized here:

1. Provide a rationale to the patient for Step 1 (e.g., "You and I have the luxury of looking back and assessing how your performance helped and hindered you to obtain what you wanted. Let's begin with the interpretations that you proposed. Let's take the first one and see how it contributed or did not contribute to you getting what you wanted, or your desired outcome") (text, pp. 143–144).
   Rule: Whenever the DO is exposed as inadequate (unattainable and/or unrealistic), it must be immediately revised and made to fit the attainable/realistic criteria before continuing with further revision (text, pp. 133–135).
2. Review each interpretation in the order that it was listed during the elicitation phase.
3. Therapist and patient assess each interpretation in terms of its relevancy and accuracy.
4. Do not disengage the cognitive interpretation from its moorings in the situation (i.e., its connection to the AO and DO).
5. Whenever the DO includes a significant partner (spouse, lover, boss, close friend, etc.) whom the therapist does *not* know, proceed with caution before concluding that the DO is unattainable. The patient must first report an SA in which he/she behaved "adaptively" with the target partner before the attainability of the DO can be determined.
6. Teach the patient to construct *action interpretations* while in stressful situations.
7. Do not revise a relevant and accurate interpretation, even when it does not contribute *directly* to DO attainment.
8. The therapist must let the patient do the work.

Review the "Patient Performance Goal for Step 1" in the text (p. 157) and summarized here:

1. The patient learns to construct relevant and accurate interpretations and to self-correct the errors.

Exercises

Following are 10 interpretation exercises. For each:

1. Answer the questions found at the end of each exercise. Each exercise will begin with a situational description and a desired outcome sentence.

2. Revise the irrelevant and inaccurate interpretations while paying close attention to the desired outcome.

3. In some instances, you will have to revise the desired outcome when it is exposed as unrealistic or unattainable.

4. After each exercise, *check your work with the criterion answers on pp. 117–121.*

Note: Before beginning, you may find it helpful to review the examples of adaptive and maladaptive interpretations in the list provided in the text (p. 118).

Interpretation Revision 1

SITUATIONAL DESCRIPTION

"I talked to one of my undergraduate students who gave a poor excuse for having missed the second test of the semester. I announced in class several times that there would be no make-up exams. The student said that his car wouldn't start on the morning of the test—that was the reason he didn't take the test. I asked why he didn't call a cab. He replied he didn't think of it. He seemed stumped when I asked what other alternatives were available (like calling me, etc.) when the car wouldn't start. He told me he just went back to sleep. Finally, I caved in and told him that he could make it up. I gave him the test, and he took it in the classroom across from my office. I slumped back in my office chair and felt like a total wimp. The limits I set don't mean anything."

DESIRED OUTCOME

"I wanted to maintain my limits of no make-up tests and tell him, 'No.' The AO did not equal the DO (AO ≠ DO)."

ELICITATION PHASE INTERPRETATIONS

1. "Nothing ever goes the way I plan it."
2. "Students are not resourceful problem solvers."
3. "I'm a loser as a professor."

a. Assess the interpretations: relevant versus irrelevant/accurate versus inaccurate (text, pp. 143–144).
   1. _____ /_____
   2. _____ /_____
   3. _____ /_____

b. Revise the interpretations to make them relevant and accurate so that they will contribute to DO attainment (if any meet criteria, leave alone).
   1. _____
   2. _____
   3. _____

c. Is an action interpretation needed here? Yes _____ No _____. If you checked "yes," then write it out: _____

_____

d. If these interpretations had been in place, do you think the patient would have been more likely to obtain the DO? Yes _____ No _____

Check your work with the criterion answers on p. 117.

Interpretation Revision 2

SITUATIONAL DESCRIPTION

"Our paperboy keeps throwing the paper on my prize rose bushes and breaking the limbs. I got up one morning before 6 A.M. to talk to him about this problem. Here he comes down the middle of the street on his bicycle, throwing papers on both sides of the street. The papers landed in ditches and bushes. Very few landed in the middle of the yards. He never slowed down to improve his aim. I asked him to stop in front of the house, and he did. I showed him my rose bushes and pointed out the damage. He seemed generally unconcerned. I asked him to be more careful and to throw my paper in the middle of the yard where there was plenty of room. He never said anything to me. He just rode off and continued throwing the papers all over the place."

DESIRED OUTCOME

"I wanted a verbal agreement from him that he would not hit my bushes again $(AO \neq DO)$."

ELICITATION PHASE INTERPRETATIONS

1. "I was upset with his behavior."
2. "I showed him where the paper had broken the limbs."
3. "He showed no concern over what he had done."
4. "He's throwing the papers in the same way."

a. Assess the interpretations: relevant versus irrelevant/accurate versus inaccurate.

1. _____ /_____
2. _____ /_____
3. _____ /_____
4. _____ /_____

b. Is an action interpretation needed here? Yes _____ No _____. If you checked "yes," then write it out: _____

_____

Check your work with the criterion answers on p. 117.

Interpretation Revision 3

SITUATIONAL DESCRIPTION

"I was talking with my supervisor Friday afternoon in the warehouse. It was 5 P.M. and quitting time. A truck had just left a load of merchandise on the loading dock. The supervisor first said that we could wait until Monday before checking the invoices. A few minutes later he told me that he wanted me to check the invoices in and then close the warehouse. I was looking at a good hour's worth of work. I told him that I had a date at 6 P.M. and couldn't do it. He insisted that I stay, saying that Monday we've got a lot of other work to do, and we need this stuff checked in. He really made me feel guilty if I didn't do it. He started talking about the good of the company and all this kind of stuff. I finally said I would do it. I closed the place up and left at 6:15 P.M. I called my date and told her about the situation. Picked her up at 8:30 P.M."

DESIRED OUTCOME

"I wanted to leave work at 5 P.M. and get ready for my date."

ELICITATION PHASE INTERPRETATIONS

1. "He ought to pick on someone else."
2. "He knows I'll do it if he insists—it's always worked in the past."
3. "I hate working at this place."

a. Assess the interpretations: relevant versus irrelevant/accurate versus inaccurate.
   1. _____ /_____
   2. _____ /_____
   3. _____ /_____

b. Revise the interpretations so that they are relevant and accurate (if any meet criteria, leave alone).
   1. _____
   2. _____
   3. _____

c. What do we call the interpretation that must be added to assure that the patient will obtain his DO? _____

d. Write out the added interpretation: _____

_____

_____

Check your work with the criterion answers on p. 118.

Interpretation Revision 4

SITUATIONAL DESCRIPTION

"I was playing bridge with my bridge club on Monday. One of the ladies always bitches at her partner. No one likes her, but she never misses our Monday bridge session. Sure enough, I got stuck with her for the first round. Everytime I bid or played a card, she had something sarcastic to say. I got so flustered that I couldn't think. Then I made more mistakes, which incited her to make even worse comments. I never said anything back to her. I remained quiet the rest of the morning."

DESIRED OUTCOME

"I wanted to tell her that she was upsetting me and making it hard for me to play my hand."

ELICITATION PHASE INTERPRETATIONS

1. "Why do I always have to get her for a partner?"
2. "Her comments make it hard for me to play my hand."
3. "The other ladies must think that I am a poor player."

a. Assess the interpretations: relevant versus irrelevant/accurate versus inaccurate (check text, p. 122, Table 6.3: *mind reading* interpretations are always rated inaccurate).

1. _____ /_____
2. _____ /_____
3. _____ /_____

b. Revise the interpretations so that they are relevant/accurate (if any meet criteria, leave alone).

1. _____
2. _____
3. _____

c. You may need to help the patient add another interpretation. Write out what this new interpretation would be: _____
_____

d. What is it called? _____

Check your work with the criterion answers on p. 118.

Interpretation Revision 5

SITUATIONAL DESCRIPTION

"I went to a party the other night. The hostess and I have known each other for a long time. When I walked in, she really looked busy. She never introduced me to anyone, which was very rude on her part. She should have known that I wanted to meet everyone. I just stood around for 45 minutes talking with the two people I knew. I finished my drink and then left."

DESIRED OUTCOME

"I wanted to meet the people I didn't know."

ELICITATION PHASE INTERPRETATIONS

1. "The hostess didn't introduce me to anyone."
2. "She should have known I wanted to meet everyone."
3. "I didn't have a good time."

a. Assess the interpretations: relevant versus irrelevant/accurate versus inaccurate.

1. _____ / _____
2. _____ / _____
3. _____ / _____

b. Revise the interpretations so that the patient could achieve the DO (if any meet criteria, leave alone).

1. _____
2. _____
3. _____

c. Would an action interpretation be helpful? Yes ____ No ____. If you answered "yes," then write the action interpretation out: _____

_____

Check your work with the criterion answers on pp. 118–119.

Interpretation Revision 6

SITUATIONAL DESCRIPTION

"I had to make a speech on Wednesday at our noon Rotary Club meeting. I always get nervous and make mistakes when I have to stand up and speak before others. I stood up, went to the podium, and gave the talk. I talked about the safety procedures airline mechanics go through when they inspect an airplane. I took the group through a mechanic's checklist of things to look for. I said 'eh' several times and stumbled once and lost my place in my notes. The club members seemed to like my talk and to be interested in what I had to say. Their questions after the talk were relevant and timely. When I went back to my seat, I received a good round of applause."

DESIRED OUTCOME

"I want to deliver my speech without any mistakes."

What is wrong with this DO? _____

_____

_____

Look at the DO the patient proposed. If you noted that it was an unrealistic DO, you would be correct (see the text, pp. 134–135). Given the patient's difficulty with making speeches, this perfectionistic DO is *not* realistic. But let it stand for the moment. We will come back to it later when we review his interpretations.

ELICITATION PHASE INTERPRETATIONS

1. "I'm nervous as hell doing this."
2. "God, I've screwed up and lost my place in my notes."
3. "I should be able to do this without any mistakes."
4. "The group liked what I had to say."

a. Assess the interpretations: relevant versus irrelevant/accurate versus inaccurate.

   1. _____ /_____
   2. _____ /_____
   3. _____ /_____
   4. _____ /_____

b. Revise the interpretations to make them relevant and accurate (if any meet criteria, leave alone).

   1. _____
   2. _____
   3. _____
   4. _____

c. Which interpretation calls into question the unrealistic nature of the DO? _____

d. Now write out a realistic DO for the patient: _____

   _____

e. How would you revise the third interpretation to describe the reality of the situation and to make it consistent with the DO? (Remember, it's got to be realistic in regard to the patient's speechmaking capability.) _____

   _____

   _____

f. Was the revised DO achieved? Yes _____ No _____

g. Why was the revised DO achieved? _____

   _____

   _____

Check your work with the criterion answers on pp. 119–120.

Interpretation Revision 7

SITUATIONAL DESCRIPTION

"I work in an office with three other people. One of them always talks loudly and is inconsiderate of the rest of us. He plays his radio loud, too. He always listens to a rock-and-roll station. Whenever he feels like it, he gets up and barges into my cubicle, sits down, and starts talking. It doesn't matter if I'm busy or not. He never asks. Tuesday morning he had been playing his radio loudly; than he came in while I was in the middle of writing a report and started talking about the Washington Redskins. I don't even like football and could care less about what the Redskins are doing. I stopped doing my work and listened to him talk for awhile. Finally he got up and left. I went back to work."

DESIRED OUTCOME

"I wish this coworker would be more considerate of me." [When asked for clarification, the patient said that she wished the guy would ask her if she had time to talk.]

ELICITATION PHASE INTERPRETATIONS

1. "My coworker is rude to me."
2. "I don't know why he treats me this way."
3. "My day is ruined."

a. Assess the interpretations: relevant versus irrelevant/accurate versus inaccurate.

1. _____ /_____
2. _____ /_____
3. _____ /_____

b. What is wrong with the DO? _____

_____

_____

c. If you don't know the answer, refer to the text, pp. 133–134. Now ask the patient to formulate a DO that *can* be achieved in light of the past and present behavior of the coworker. Write it out: _____

_____

_____

_____

d. Now go back to step *a* and complete your assessment of interpretations 2 and 3. What type of interpretation must be added to increase the likelihood that the reformulated DO will be obtained? _____

e. Write out the added interpretation from *d*. _____

_____

_____

Check your work with the criterion answers on p. 120.

Interpretation Revision 8

SITUATIONAL DESCRIPTION

"My older brother and I were watching a ball game on Saturday. Out of the blue he started making nasty comments about my girlfriend. He said I only date losers. I first thought he was kidding, but then I realized that something more was going on here. He was really serious. I told him, 'Shut up, you are full of it!' Then I told him he was a poor excuse for a brother and said some other really bad things about his character. Everytime he said something else, I laid into him again about all his failures. He looked hurt, got up, and left the room. We haven't spoken for two days."

DESIRED OUTCOME

"I wanted to hurt my brother as much as I could." [Review the text, pp. 136–138. In this case, the therapist was uncomfortable with the DO, and the patient looked somewhat sad in going through the SA.]

ELICITATION PHASE INTERPRETATIONS

1. "My brother is really on my case."
2. "I want to hurt him bad and remind him of all the things he has failed at."

a. How would you respond to a patient if his/her DO left you feeling uncomfortable? Remember, the goal at this point is to get to the heart of why the patient, in this case, wants to hurt his brother. The component of *having been hurt* is not evident in the interpretations nor in the DO. Think through your strategy carefully and write out what you would say to this patient about his DO: _____

_____

_____

_____

b. Formulate a revised DO: _____

_____

_____

c. Revise the interpretations using the reformulated DO:
   1. _____
   2. _____

Note: This type of SA is always difficult to manage. The goal is to get to the "kernel of hurt" that is driving the anger and the motive to retaliate. Once the hurt is exposed, the theme of the revised DO must be to help the patient inquire why the perpetrator wants to inflict the pain. Otherwise, the anger and vengeance DO will have a circular effect (e.g., "We have not spoken for two days") and the conflict will continue unresolved.

Check your work with the criterion answers on pp. 120–121.

Interpretation Revision 9

SITUATIONAL DESCRIPTION

"I told my husband that I wanted to rearrange the living room furniture by moving the sofa and loveseat around and placing the coffee table in the far corner of the room, adjacent to the love seat. He said to me: 'That's the stupidest thing I ever heard of. Only you would come up with such a plan.' He also told me that all my ideas were stupid and lousy and that I don't have a creative bone in my body. I replied that he never likes anything I try to do. I started crying and went to the bedroom and slammed the door."

DESIRED OUTCOME

"I wanted my husband to help me move the furniture."

ELICITATION PHASE INTERPRETATIONS

    1. "My husband never likes anything I want to do."
    2. "I can't do anything right."
    3. "Why do I ever try to do anything?"

  a. Assess the interpretations: relevant versus irrelevant/accurate versus inaccurate.
    1. _____ /_____
    2. _____ /_____
    3. _____ /_____

  b. Is a DO revision necessary? If so, write out a revised DO: _____
    _____
    _____

  c. Revise the interpretations to make them relevant and accurate so that they will increase the possibility of achieving the DO. (If any meet criteria, leave alone.)
    1. _____
    2. _____
    3. _____

d. Is an action interpretation needed here? Yes _____ No _____

e. If you answered "yes," then write out the action interpretation that is needed or note which of your revised interpretations serves this purpose: _____

_____

_____

Check your work with the criterion answers on p. 121.

Interpretation Revision 10

SITUATIONAL DESCRIPTION

"I drove my car to the gas station to get a state inspection done. The owner of the station told me that I was next in line. He said my wait would be about 30 minutes. I have a late model Honda, so I didn't expect the mechanic to find anything wrong. While sitting in the waiting area, I saw another car drive up, a Lincoln Town Car, and the gas station manager allowed him to put his car ahead of mine. I got up and went to the manager and told him that he said I was next in line. I also said that I didn't want to be bumped back a slot because I had to get to the office. The owner mumbled something under his breath and then put my car back in line where it was. I got the inspection done, paid cash, and was out in about 30 minutes."

DESIRED OUTCOME

"I wanted to get the state inspection and remain next in line."

ELICITATION PHASE INTERPRETATIONS

1. "The inspection ought to be finished in 30 minutes."
2. "The owner has bumped me back a car."
3. "I've got to tell the manager that I want my car put back next in line."

a. Assess the interpretations: relevant or irrelevant/accurate or inaccurate.

1. _____ / _____

2. _____ / _____

3. _____ / _____

b. What characteristics of the interpretations led directly to the achievement of the DO? Write it out: _____

_____

_____

Check your work with the criterion answers on p. 121.

Criterion Answers for Step 1 Remediation Exercises

Interpretation Revision 1

a. Assess interpretations:

1. Irrelevant/inaccurate: If an interpretation is irrelevant (i.e., not anchored in the situation-at-hand), it cannot be accurate (describe what is going on in the situation). Be on the lookout for *adverbs* in the interpretation sentences; in most instances, adverbs signal irrelevant interpretations.
2. Irrelevant/inaccurate: This is a generalization that disengages the interpretation from the problem. Had the interpretation been stated, "This student is not a resourceful problem solver," it would have been a relevant and accurate interpretation.
3. Irrelevant/inaccurate: Again, this interpretation does not address the problem-at-hand, nor does it help the professor maintain the limits he announced on make-ups.

b. Revise interpretations:

1. "The student's excuse is not acceptable to me."
2. "The student is a poor problem solver."
3. "I've got to tell the student no (action interpretation)."

c. Yes: "I've got to tell the student no."
d. Yes. Note that interpretations 1 and 3 must be discarded, while 2 is revised to described this particular student. When the revision process is complete, the professor is anchored in the situation and connected to his original plan of allowing no make-up tests.

Interpretation Revision 2

a. Assess interpretations:

1. Relevant/accurate.
2. Relevant/accurate.
3. Relevant/accurate.
4. Relevant/accurate.

b. Revise interpretations:

Yes. "I must ask him to verbally agree that he will not hit my bushes again."

Note. It is obvious that the patient has a very difficult situation on his hands. The paperboy might agree verbally but then keep throwing the papers in the rose bushes. However, we won't know the outcome until the patient obtains his DO by getting a verbal agreement from the paperboy in this situation.

Interpretation Revision 3

a. Assess interpretations:

1. Irrelevant/inaccurate.
2. Irrelevant/inaccurate: Note the adverb "always."
3. Irrelevant/inaccurate.

b. Revise interpretations:

1. "I don't want to stay late."
2. "The invoice check can wait until Monday."
3. "My supervisor is not going to change his mind easily."

Note: Proceed with caution in situations like this and do not reflexively encourage an action read that would lead to negative work outcomes. The best rule-of-thumb is to follow the patient's lead, or at least question the patient about the consequences of saying no to the boss.

c. Action interpretation.
d. "I've got to tell him that he'll have to find someone else to check the invoices."

Interpretation Revision 4

a. Assess interpretations:

1. Irrelevant/inaccurate.
2. Relevant/accurate.
3. Irrelevant/inaccurate: this is a "mind read interpretation," and it is always rated irrelevant/inaccurate. The rule here is the following: *If you don't ask what another person is thinking, you don't know!*

b. Revise interpretations:

1. "I don't like playing with this bridge partner."
2. Meets criterion.
3. "She says something sarcastic about everything I do" (action interpretation).

c. "I've got to tell her that her negative comments make it difficult for me to play my hand."

d. Action interpretation.

Interpretation Revision 5

a. Assess interpretations:

1. Relevant/accurate.
2. Irrelevant/inaccurate: mind-reading interpretation.
3. Relevant/accurate.

  b. Revise interpretations:

    1. Meets criterion.

    2. "I've got to ask the hostess to introduce me when she gets the chance" (action interpretation).

    Note. The original interpretation is a frequent one among chronic patients who often think others ought to know what they want/need even though they do not verbalize anything.

    3. Meets criterion.

  c. Yes.

  Note. If the patient had inserted an action read in place of interpretation 2, she might have achieved her DO. It is obvious that if she had met the people she didn't know, the party would have been more fun.

Interpretation Revision 6

  a. Assess interpretations:

    1. Relevant/accurate.

    2. Relevant/accurate.

    3. Relevant/inaccurate: Notice that the interpretation is anchored in the event, but it does not describe accurately what is going on in the situation. The fact that the patient *did* make mistakes means that the interpretation is inaccurate. The patient must deal with the fact that he cannot realistically produce what he wants in the situation. At this point, the interpretation will need to be revised.

    4. Relevant/accurate.

  b. Revise interpretations:

    1. Meets criterion.

    2. Meets criterion.

    3. "I've made a mistake, but I recovered okay."

    Note: Here the clinician must step in and question the patient about the realistic nature of his DO. As stated above, the issue here is the following: You are *not* going to make a perfect speech, so what is a realistic DO for you in this situation?

    4. Meets criterion.

  c. Interpretation 3.

  d. *Revised DO:* "I want to complete my speech to the Rotary Club."

  e. "I've made a mistake, but I recovered okay."

  f. Yes.

  g. "Because I stayed grounded in the situation and finished my speech."

Note: Revising DOs in the remediation phase takes practice. Extensive practice in this area is provided at CBASP training workshops and through the continued assistance of supervisory feedback following the workshop.

Interpretation Revision 7

a. Assess interpretations:

  1. Relevant/accurate.
  2. Relevant/inaccurate: The fact that the coworker is *not* considerate of his office mates calls into question the *attainability* of the DO from the outset. *The DO must be revised before going any further.*
  3. Irrelevant/inaccurate: Must be revised or discarded.

b. The DO is *unattainable*; the patient must create a DO that is within *his* power to attain.

c. *Revised DO:* "I want to tell my coworker that I'm busy and cannot talk now."

d. An action interpretation replaces interpretation 2. Interpretation 3 can be discarded. It does not contribute to DO attainment.

e. "I've got to tell my coworker that I'm busy and cannot talk now.

Note: Are you feeling a little more comfortable now with DO revision? Teaching patients that they cannot "put square pegs in round holes"—that they cannot ask reality to be other than what it is—is the basic rationale for DO revision.

Interpretation Revision 8

a. Assess interpretations:

> THERAPIST: I'm uncomfortable with your DO, and you look somewhat sad in telling me about the event.
>
> PATIENT: It was not good.
>
> THERAPIST: Why not?
>
> PATIENT: He really hurt me.
>
> THERAPIST: I don't see any of this expressed in your DO.
>
> PATIENT: What do you mean?
>
> THERAPIST: Your DO doesn't reflect that your goal was to let him know how badly he had hurt you.
>
> PATIENT: If I had done that, we might have avoided the way it ended up.
>
> THERAPIST: Let's go back and rework the situation using a DO that lets your brother know how badly he has hurt you.

b. *Revised DO:* "I want to let my brother know how much he has hurt me."

   c. Revise interpretations:

      1. "My brother is really on my case."
      2. "I've got to let him know he's leaning on me" (action interpretation).

Interpretation Revision 9

   a. Assess interpretations:

      1. Irrelevant/inaccurate.
      2. Irrelevant/inaccurate.
      3. Irrelevant/inaccurate.

   b. Yes. "I want to tell my husband he's hurt me badly by his comments."
   c. Revise interpretations:

      1. "My husband is angry, and I don't know why."
      2. "He's really hurt me with his comments."
      3. "I've got to ask why he hurt me in this way."

      Note: Relevant and accurate interpretations serve to ground patients and put them in an optimal position to deal with the stress-at-hand—in this case, a hostile response from the husband.

   d. Yes.
   e. "I've got to ask why he hurt me in this way."

Interpretation Revision 10

   a. Assess interpretations:

      1. Relevant/accurate.
      2. Relevant/accurate.
      3. Relevant/accurate.

   b. The interpretations described the unfolding events accurately and, in so doing, kept the patient grounded and knowing what she had to do when she lost her place in line.

STEP 2: REMEDIATION OF BEHAVIOR

SECTION A
Targeting the Behaviors Needed to Obtain the Desired Outcome

The exercises in Section A provide practice in targeting the behaviors that are required to obtain the DO. Patients learn two things through their SA work: (1) to keep the DO clearly in mind throughout a situation; and (2) to take effective action in order to obtain the DO. Formulating *action interpretations* during an interaction requires that one use both of the above skills.

Section B exercises provide practice in planning in-session training to teach the requisite behavioral skills. Sometimes it is not what patients *do* that sabotages their efforts, it is *the way* they go about doing it. People communicate with each other employing various interpersonal styles. Each style has a "stimulus value" for others; each style "pulls" certain automatic responses out of others. The responses may be positive-facilitative or negative-rejecting, or they may fall somewhere on a continuum between the two poles. More often than not, chronically depressed adults pull negative-rejecting reactions from others. In order to help patients elicit more positive responses, interpersonal feedback about communication style, training, and practice are administered during therapy sessions.

Now we turn to the Section A exercises involved in Step 2 of the remediation process.

Review

Review the "Therapist Rules for Administering Step 2" in the text (pp. 157–161) and summarized here:

1. Teach patients that their cognitive interpretations are functionally related to their situational behavior.
2. Pinpoint the behaviors that contribute directly to DO achievement.
3. Target the behaviors that need to be modified, as well as those that need to be added, in order to obtain the DO.
4. Teach new behavioral skills, *but only after the SA has been completed.*
5. Teach patients to evaluate their situational behavior in light of the DO and to self-correct the problem behaviors.

Review the "Patient Performance Goals for Step 2" in the text (p. 161) and summarized here:

1. Patient learns to evaluate his/her situational behavior and to self-correct the errors.
2. Patient learns the necessary behavioral skills that lead to DO attainment.

Exercises

Following are 10 remediation targeting exercises. For each:

1. Review the revised SA interpretations and DOs in each exercise and pinpoint the behavior(s) that will be needed to obtain the DO.
2. Each exercise parallels the situational content in the exercise in the previous section; however, the interpretations in this section are all relevant and accurate.
3. After each exercise, *check your work with the criterion answers on p. 128.*

Remediation Targeting 1

INTERPRETATIONS

1. "The student's excuse is not acceptable to me."
2. "The student is a poor problem solver."
3. "I've got to tell the student that he cannot take a make-up exam."

DESIRED OUTCOME

"I want to maintain my limits of no make-up exams."

REQUIRED BEHAVIOR

What behavior is required for DO attainment?: _____

_____

Check your work with the criterion answer on p. 128.

Remediation Targeting 2

INTERPRETATIONS

1. "I was upset with the careless way he threw the newspapers."
2. "I showed him where the paper had broken my rosebushes."
3. "He showed no concern over what he had done."
4. "I must ask him to agree that he will not hit my bushes again."

DESIRED OUTCOME

"I wanted a verbal agreement that he would not hit my bushes again."

REQUIRED BEHAVIOR

What behavior is required for DO attainment?: _____

_____

Check your work with the criterion answer on p. 128.

Remediation Targeting 3

INTERPRETATIONS

1. "I don't want to stay late to check the invoices."
2. "Checking the invoices can wait until Monday."
3. "I've got to tell my boss that he'll have to find someone else to do this job."

DESIRED OUTCOME

"I want to leave work at 5 P.M. and get ready for my date.

REQUIRED BEHAVIOR

What behavior is required for DO attainment?: _____

_____

Check your work with the criterion answer on p. 128.

Remediation Targeting 4

INTERPRETATIONS

1. "I don't like playing with this bridge partner."
2. "Her comments make it hard for me to play my hand."
3. "I've got to tell her that her negative comments make it difficult for me to play my hand."

DESIRED OUTCOME

"I want to tell her that she is upsetting me and making it hard for me to play my hand."

REQUIRED BEHAVIOR

What behavior is required for DO attainment?: _____

_____

Check your work with the criterion answer on p. 128.

Remediation Targeting 5

INTERPRETATIONS

1. "The hostess didn't introduce me to anyone."
2. "I've got to ask the hostess to introduce me around when she gets the chance."

DESIRED OUTCOME

"I want to meet the people I don't know."

REQUIRED BEHAVIOR

What behavior is required for DO attainment?: _____

_____

Check your work with the criterion answer on p. 128.

Remediation Targeting 6

INTERPRETATIONS

1. "I'm nervous as hell giving this speech."
2. "God, I've screwed up and lost my place in my notes."
3. "I've made a mistake, but I recovered okay."
4. "The group liked what I had to say."

DESIRED OUTCOME

"I want to complete my speech to the Rotary Club."

REQUIRED BEHAVIOR

What behavior is required for DO attainment?: _____

_____

Check your work with the criterion answer on p. 128.

Remediation Targeting 7

INTERPRETATIONS

1. "My coworker is rude to me."
2. "I've got to tell my coworker that I'm busy and can't talk now."

DESIRED OUTCOME

"Tell my coworker that I'm busy and can't talk now."

REQUIRED BEHAVIOR

What behavior is required for DO attainment?: _____

_____

Check your work with the criterion answer on p. 128.

Remediation Targeting 8

INTERPRETATIONS

1. "My brother is really on my case about my girlfriend."
2. "I've got to let him know he leaning on me too hard."

DESIRED OUTCOME

"I want to let my brother know that he is leaning on me too hard."

REQUIRED BEHAVIOR

What behavior is required for DO attainment?: _____

_____

Check your work with the criterion answer on p. 128.

Remediation Targeting 9

INTERPRETATIONS

1. "My husband is angry at me, and I don't know why."
2. "He's really hurt me with his comments."
3. "I've got to ask him why he's hurt me this way."

DESIRED OUTCOME

"I want to ask my husband why he wanted to hurt me this way."

REQUIRED BEHAVIOR

What behavior is required for DO attainment?: _____

_____

Check your work with the criterion answer on p. 128.

Remediation Targeting 10

INTERPRETATIONS

1. "The inspection ought to be finished in 30 minutes."
2. "The manager has let someone in line ahead of me."
3. "I've got to tell the manager that I want my car put back in line."

DESIRED OUTCOME

"I want the state inspection completed and to maintain my place in line."

REQUIRED BEHAVIOR

What behavior is required for DO attainment?: _____

_____

Check your work with the criterion answer on p. 128.

Note: Every behavior in these exercises involved some form of assertive action. Teaching patients to maintain their sights on what they want (the DO) and then to behave in ways that are likely to achieve it are some of the basic goals of SA. Being able to generate action interpretations while in the heat of the situation is a skill that requires repeated practice. Action interpretations can be generated easily as long as the individual remains cognizant of his/her DO.

Criterion Answers for Step 2, Section A, Remediation Exercises

Remediation Targeting 1

Setting verbal limits on the student in a calm, direct manner.

Remediation Targeting 2

Requesting a verbal agreement.

Remediation Targeting 3

Telling the supervisor that he will have to find someone else to check the invoices.

Remediation Targeting 4

Telling the bridge partner that her comments are making it difficult for me to play.

Remediation Targeting 5

Telling the hostess that I would like to be introduced to the people I don't know.

Remediation Targeting 6

Sustaining and focusing my behavior until the speech is finished.

Remediation Targeting 7

Telling coworker that I'm busy now and cannot talk.

Remediation Targeting 8

Telling brother that he has hurt me with his remarks about my girlfriend.

Remediation Targeting 9

Asking husband why he wants to hurt me by his comments.

Remediation Targeting 10

Telling the manager to put my car back in its original place in line.

SECTION B
Constructing Training Plans to Teach Needed Interpersonal Skills

As noted earlier, patients often create the interpersonal problems they complain about because of their stylistic communication patterns. Speaking in a whiny tone of voice, using invasive or disruptive speech that creates anger reactions, talking in a vague or evasive manner that leaves the interactant confused and unsure about what the person has said, engaging in sexual gestures or innuendoes that are situationally inappropriate, dressing in a sloppy or unkept manner that makes others withdraw or be nonresponsive—the list of possible interpersonal problems is endless. However, the negative consequences for these varied behaviors are similar: *interpersonal rejection*! Teaching patients to modify these disruptive mannerisms enhances the quality of their interpersonal encounters and facilitates DO achievement.

I must state one caveat before continuing. Interpersonal training of the type covered in this section requires that therapists first become aware of their own stimulus value. Educating CBASP therapists about their stimulus value is undertaken in small group exercises during CBASP workshops and continues during intensive supervision that leads to CBASP certification. An old adage describes our approach to interpersonal behavioral training: *"It takes one to know one."* Once CBASP therapists become aware of their own stimulus impact on others, then—and only then—are they ready to demonstrate the patient's stimulus value on themselves.

Review

Review Chapters Eight (pp. 167–195) and Thirteen (pp. 256–274) in the text before completing the Section B exercises. In summary:

1. Chapter Eight describes how CBASP therapists use disciplined personal involvement as one vehicle to modify interpersonal behavior.
2. Dealing with patient crises is the subject of Chapter Thirteen. In most cases, clinicians can facilitate change by using their personal reactions as consequences to modify in-session crisis behavior.

Exercises

Following are 10 remediation training exercises. For each:

1. Identify four different types of maladaptive interpersonal behavior. Then construct a remedial training plan for the problem behavior in each scenario.
2. *Note:* Four types of maladaptive interpersonal behavior that require remediation following the completion of the SA include:

   a. *Lack of empathy:* focusing on the literal content of the conversation and not on the other person's affective agenda; failure to acknowledge the other person's expressed emotions; failure to observe visual and other nonverbal channels of communication by which to gather information about affect and intent.

b. *Hostile speech patterns/demeanor*: strident/hostile tone of voice or actual hostile verbalizations (usually framed in global, not specific, terms); changing subject abruptly without regard for the other person; talking too fast.

c. *Overly controlling interpersonal behavior*: excessive attempts to talk for others, tell others what they are thinking, or organize the behavior of others; overt control of conversations; impulsively helping others even before they request assistance; keeping others at a distance by trying to control their behavior.

d. *Lack of assertive behavior*: not making concise, declarative "I" statements of wants, needs, situational concerns, and so on; excessive elaboration, explanations, or justification of one's point; not maintaining eye contact with the person spoken to; voice tone too low/soft to be heard; speaking in a whining or pleading voice; refusing to make a decision because of needing more information.

3. Each scenario presents one type of maladaptive interpersonal behavior.
4. First, label the maladaptive type of behavior in the scenario (use the list above).
5. Next, write out a description of your behavioral training plan, detailing how you would modify the behavior. A simple plan is always best.

Note: These interpersonal skills will be identified and addressed during Step 2 of the remediation phase. When more intensive work and practice is required, this activity should be carried out *after* the SA has been completed (during the behavioral skill training/rehearsal period).

After completing each exercise, *check your work with the criterion answers on pp. 135–139.*

Remediation Training 1 (Male Therapist/Male Patient)

The clinician enters the therapy room a few minutes after the receptionist has seated the patient. He had obviously been running, for he is panting, sweating, and out of breath. He collapses in his chair saying, "Whew! Sorry I'm late. I ran all the way from the subway exit." The patient looks at his watch and replies, "I've been waiting for 3 minutes."

a. Type of maladaptive behavior: _____

b. Behavioral training plan: _____

_____

_____

Check your work with the criterion answers on p. 135.

Remediation Training 2 (Male Therapist/Female Patient)

MARY: Dr. Smith, I been seeing you for 4 weeks now. You always see me at the end of your day, and you've just got to be tired of listening to people's complaints. Why don't we end this session early so you can go home to your family and get some rest. It would be all right with me if we stopped early.

DR. SMITH: Mary, I'm feeling fine, and I'm not really tired. I don't want to end your session early.

MARY: Well, if you're not going to take care of yourself, then I'll have to do it for you. Give yourself a break and let's stop early.

a. Type of maladaptive behavior: _____

b. Behavioral training plan: _____

_____

_____

Check your work with the criterion answers on p. 135.

Remediation Training 3 (Male Therapist/Male Patient)

"I hate my boss. I can't think of one good characteristic he possesses. Everything he says is irrelevant or wrong. No one in the company has any respect for him. I can't understand how he got to be an executive in this company. I've never heard of one thing he has done well. I went to Sears yesterday, and couldn't find anyone to wait on me. When I finally ran down a salesman—and I had to *find* him—he was unable to tell me what I wanted to know. Incompetence is everywhere. I'm not going to vote this year because of the bums who are running. No wonder the country is going to the dogs. God, what a screwed up world we live in."

a. Type of maladaptive behavior: _____

b. Behavioral training plan: _____

_____

_____

Check your work with the criterion answers on pp. 135–136.

Remediation Training 4 (Male Therapist/Male Patient)

PATIENT: I would really like for my wife to stop criticizing me in front of others. She does it whenever company comes over, when we go to someone's house or to a party with friends. She even started talking about my faults at a Little League game the other night, while we were sitting in the stands with several other parents.

THERAPIST: What have you said to her about this?

PATIENT: I told her that other husbands' wives don't talk about their spouses this way. I've pointed out how happy other couples are. Fred and Judy are a case in point. Judy never says an unkind word about Fred. We have been with them on a number of occasions, and they hardly ever disagree. I don't see how people live that way. It's certainly not the way we live. I think it would be nice if wives said only nice things about their husbands.

a. Type of maladaptive behavior: _____

b. Behavioral training plan: _____

_____

_____

Check your work with the criterion answers on p. 136.

Remediation Training 5 (Male Therapist/Female Patient)

PATIENT: (*Patient looks at the floor; refuses to make eye contact with the therapist, voice very soft; shoulders droop and her general posture suggests abasement and low self-esteem; her general demeanor is tentative; facial features express fear/foreboding.*) I apologize for being late to my appointment this afternoon. My bus was late, and there was nothing I could do about it.

THERAPIST: I'm just glad you made it. It's good to see you.

PATIENT: I don't see how you can say this. I mean, about how good it is to see me. No one else has ever said that to me (*voice drifting off, gaze still on the floor*). My husband is never glad to see me. When I come around, he looks at me in a disgusted way. I think I'd better quit therapy before I disgust you too. There's no way you will want to see me as a patient after you get to know me.

a. Type of maladaptive behavior: _____

b. Behavioral training plan: _____

_____

_____

Check your work with the criterion answers on pp. 136–137.

Remediation Training 6 (Female Therapist/Female Patient)

THERAPIST: My mother locked me out of the house when I was 16 years old and had come home late from a date. I knocked on the front door and asked her to let me in. She screamed from inside the house: "Whores can't sleep in my house! Go find another man's bed to sleep in." I had to call a friend and ask if I could sleep over. The next morning I went back home and found the door open. This kind of bizarre incident with my mother was not unusual. [The clinician's personal disclosure was accompanied by misty eyes and a pained expression on her face.]

PATIENT: My mother was meaner than your mother. She wouldn't have opened the door the next morning. You had it easy.

a. Type of maladaptive behavior: _____

b. Behavioral training plan: _____

_____

_____

Check your work with the criterion answers on p. 137.

Remediation Training 7 (Female Therapist/Female Patient)

"You always ask too much of me. I can't do what you want. This therapy stuff is a waste of my time and money. I don't even think you will be able to help me. Sorry I ever decided to see you in the first place. You're just like my mother, you ask impossible things of me!"

a. Type of maladaptive behavior: _____

b. Behavioral training plan: _____

_____

_____

Check your work with the criterion answers on p. 137.

Remediation Training 8 (Male Therapist/Female Patient)

PATIENT: I brought you some cake. Made it this morning, just for you. I hope you like it.

THERAPIST: You have been very thoughtful. Last week you brought me food, and the week before that you agreed to shift your appointment to another day because of my out-of-town meeting.

PATIENT: I just like to be helpful and to try to do thoughtful things for other people. Is there anything else I can do for you? I want you to let me know whenever I can help you out. Will you do that for me?

a. Type of maladaptive behavior: _____

b. Behavioral training plan: _____

_____

_____

Check your work with the criterion answers on pp. 137–138.

Remediation Training 9 (Female Therapist/Female Patient)

"My dad came over to talk to me this weekend about a legal matter that he was concerned about. He didn't look pleased when I opened the door and invited him in. My husband spoke to him briefly, then went downstairs to work in his basement shop. I was in the middle of fixing dinner, so I asked Dad to come back to the kitchen and sit with me while I cut up vegetables to cook. I was not sure how to start the conversation about the legal issue. Guess I just avoided it by doing other things. My friend called me, and we talked about the party she and I were having next Saturday night. Her child cut his finger and came running in the house, and she had to go tend to him so she got off the phone. I remembered that I had not finished sewing the hem of my skirt, so I went to get it and finish the sewing while the vegetables were cooking. Dad just sat there, and he and I didn't say very much."

a. Type of maladaptive behavior: _____

b. Behavioral training plan: _____

_____

_____

Check your work with the criterion answers on p. 138.

Remediation Training 10 (Male Therapist/Female Patient)

THERAPIST: For the past few weeks you have presented SAs in which you have done everything right and obtained your DO. Yet you stay depressed. Your life seems "okay," yet I get the feeling that there are areas of your life where things are not going so well. What about this? Am I right?

PATIENT: Well, I do have some real problems, but I don't want to burden you with them. You seem to have enough on your plate already with your sick child and the research grant you are working on. If I began to get into some of the stuff going on between me and my husband, then that would be another burden you would have to bear. I don't want to do this to you—to become another problem for you. I like it better when I can make things easy on you.

a. Type of maladaptive behavior: _____

b. Behavioral training plan: _____

_____

_____

Check your work with the criterion answers on pp. 138–139.

Criterion Answers for Step 2, Section B, Remediation Exercises

Remediation Training 1

a. Lack of empathy.

b. Behavioral training plan:

1. Focus patient's attention on therapist's physical condition and have patient describe it (panting, sweating, out of breath).

2. Focus patient's attention on *content* of what therapist has just said ("I'm sorry that I am late, I've been running all the way").

3. Focus patient's attention on the *intent* of the verbal comments (I did not want to be late for our appointment).

4. *Ask the patient:* "Why do you think I said this to you when I first came in?"

5. *Goal of the training plan:* To help the patient become aware of the therapist's stimulus signals, to learn to read them correctly, and to respond in an empathic manner.

Remediation Training 2

a. Maladaptive behavior: overly controlling interpersonal behavior.

b. Behavioral training plan:

1. Focus patient's attention on the clinician's response to the patient's original statement about stopping early.

2. Ask the patient to repeat what was said.

3. Ask the patient *why* it is difficult to believe what the therapist said. *Note:* Don't be put off by intellectual reasons such as, "Yes, you said this, *but* . . . "). The problem here is that *the therapist's comments do not yet inform the patient's thinking and therefore her behavior.*

4. *Goal of the training plan:* Maintain the focus on what actually happened. The patient cannot yet take the clinician's comments seriously. The interpersonal consequence for the therapist is to feel written off by the patient. The patient must receive this feedback. Teaching patients to listen to others and then to take what they say seriously is one way to modify overly controlling interpersonal patterns.

Remediation Training 3

a. Maladaptive behavior: hostile speech patterns/demeanor.

b. Behavioral training plan:

1. Say to the patient: "Let's review what you just said to me. Please summarize it for me." Allow the individual to recall and restate the negative ravings. Not infrequently, patients are not able to recall what they have just said. A reminder or two from the clinician is acceptable.

2. Focus the patient's attention on the interpersonal *consequences* these ravings have

on the therapist. A question like this is often effective: "What effect do you think these comments have just had on me?" The patient is unlikely to know.

3. Provide "consequation" feedback. For example: "It makes me want to tune you out." or "I feel like you just want to bitch and you don't care what my reactions are."

4. Ask the question, "Why do you want to have these effects on me?" *Note*: Don't be deflected by such comments as, "I didn't mean to do this," and the like. Maintain the focus on the actual behavior and the actual consequences that have just occurred.

5. *Goal of the training plan*: Educate the patient as to his/her stimulus value in such moments. Ultimately the patient must make a choice: Do I want to have this effect, or another?

Remediation Training 4

a. Maladaptive behavior: lack of assertive behavior.
b. Behavioral training plan:

1. Ask the patient to construct one declarative sentence (an "I want" type of sentence) specifying what he wants his wife to do.

2. Once the desired outcome is stated in a declarative manner, then role play the interaction between husband and wife, with the therapist taking the wife's role.

3. *Goal of the training plan*: Let the husband practice talking in declarative sentences until he can articulate the DO in a direct and lucid manner. Provide interpersonal feedback throughout the practice trials.

Remediation Training 5

a. Maladaptive behavior: lack of assertive behavior.
b. Behavioral training plan:

1. Ask the patient, "How do you know that I won't want to see you once I get to know you?" Focus the patient's attention on her expectancies of the clinician. Once the rejection expectancies are made explicit, shift the attention to another area.

2. Ask the patient, "How could you know how I feel about you?" Help the patient talk about how we gain knowledge about the way others feel and think about us: by (1) observing their nonverbal cues, (2) listening to what they say about us, and (3) asking another person how he/she feels about us. Now, shift the attention to the therapist's appearance.

3. Say to the patient the following: "I want you to look me over—take your time—and tell me what you see that would indicate how I feel about you." *Note*: Give the patient sufficient time to do this—it will likely be a novel and frightening interpersonal request. Confirm any correct observations, such as "you are making eye contact with me," "you are smiling at me," "you've said supportive things to me," and so on.

4. *Goal of the training plan*: The patient gains facility in recognizing communication cues and responding appropriately to them. *Note:* If a patient cannot make any positive observations, then the practitioner may have to suggest several possibilities. This exercise should be repeated at the beginning of therapy sessions until the negative expectancies become a non-issue for the patient.

Remediation Training 6

a. Maladaptive behavior: lack of empathy.
b. Behavioral training plan:

1. Focus the patient's attention on the therapist's nonverbal expressions of sadness and pain. Ask the patient to describe these nonverbal behaviors.
2. Inquire what emotional reactions or memories the patient had during the clinician's disclosure. Ask the patient to articulate these and to attend to the emotions that were present.
3. Ask the patient to articulate what feelings the therapist must have been experiencing when she told her story about her mother's behavior.
4. Discuss the concept of *empathy* and how it can be used to strengthen interpersonal relationships. End the discussion by reviewing the patient's initial competitive reaction and compare and contrast this with the consequences that usually follow empathic responses.
5. *Goal for the training plan*: The patient is able to listen to, and remained focused on, the therapist's description of a personal experience, and respond appropriately.

Remediation Training 7

a. Maladaptive behavior: hostile speech patterns/demeanor.
b. Behavioral training plan:

1. Ask the patient, "What did your mother do when you reacted to her the way you just reacted to me?" (The mother probably responded in a hostile manner and a fight ensued.)
2. Focus the patient's attention on the clinician's positive reaction to this harsh outburst by saying something like, "Describe how I just reacted to you."
3. *Goal of the training plan*: Help the patient discriminate between the negative reactions of the mother and the clinician's positive-facilitative reaction. The final step here involves a discussion of the implications of having a relationship with someone whose behavior is different from the mother's.

Remediation Training 8

a. Maladaptive behavior: overcontrolling interpersonal behavior.
b. Behavioral training plan:

1. Ask the patient, "Have you ever thought about my reactions to your helping behavior? Why don't you ask me what they are?" The therapist is shifting the attention from the patient to himself. The consequences of the patient's behavior are going to be made explicit. The following dialogue, in general, takes place:

THERAPIST: I feel intimidated by what you do for me.

PATIENT: I don't understand.

THERAPIST: Obviously, I can't reciprocate your many considerations, so I always feel that I'm "one down" to you.

PATIENT: But that's not what I want to do to you. I don't want to make you feel this way.

THERAPIST: But you *do* make me feel this way. I really believe you, though, that this is not how you want to make me feel.

PATIENT: You're right.

THERAPIST: Then how could you avoid doing this to me in the future?

2. *Goal of the training plan:* By focusing the patient on the consequences of her behavior, the practitioner can assist her to become aware of her stimulus value and teach her to "ask" before impulsively assisting others.

Remediation Training 9

a. Maladaptive behavior: lack of assertive behavior.
b. Behavioral training plan:

1. Help the patient formulate a DO for this situation by answering the question, "How did you want this situation to come out?" The patient would probably say that she wanted to discuss the legal matter her dad was concerned about.
2. Ask the patient, "How could you arrange your activities so that you could accomplish this goal?" Planning the activities, using a pencil and paper, may be necessary.
3. *Goal of the training plan:* Construct a DO and then review an activity plan. An activity plan is necessary if the patient is to obtain the DO.

Remediation Training 10

a. Maladaptive behavior: interpersonal overcontrol pattern.
b. Behavioral training plan:

1. Ask the patient, "How do you know that talking about your problems places a burden on me?" The goal here is to have the patient learn to ask questions and not "mind read" the clinician.
2. The credibility of the therapist's answer that he is not burdened by her problems may become an issue (she may find it difficult to take what the therapist says seriously). The focus is on *why* it is hard to believe what the practitioner says.

3. Once the "why issue" has been exposed, the therapist must help the patient learn to take him seriously, and then transfer this new found skill to her other relationships. In all probability, the patient has not had interpersonal experiences wherein she felt that what she said had been taken seriously. The clinician has the opportunity to be one of the first persons to take the patient seriously—but then he must make certain the patient recognizes what is taking place in such moments. With such patients, being taken seriously and learning to take the therapist seriously will remain an important goal issue throughout treatment.

4. *Goal of the training plan*: The goal here is to teach the patient to deal realistically with the therapist and, in so doing, to take better care of herself. This problem is similar to several other scenarios. Once again, the patient is "taking care" of the therapist. The therapist will then assist her to talk about the "burden" she perceives she places on others, and teach her not to deal with an unrealistic person who does not exist.

STEP 3: WRAP-UP AND SUMMARY OF SA

Review

Review the "Therapist Rules for Administering Step 3" in the text (pp. 162–163) and summarized here:

1. Therapist should sit back and allow the patient to assess what he/she has just learned in SA.
2. Allow the patient to provide the summary review first.
3. If an important part(s) of the SA has been overlooked, *then, and only then,* should these behaviors be called to the patient's attention.

Review the "Patient Performance Goal for Step 3" in the text (p. 163) and summarized here:

1. The patient must learn to focus on relevant components of the SA remediation exercise that have led to DO attainment.

Exercises

1. *Rank order* the following Wrap-up/Summary statements taken from five chronically depressed patients beginning with *highest quality statement* and ending with the lowest. The key discriminating variable here is the degree to which patients are aware of the fact that their behavior has specific consequences in the environment (i.e., the degree to which the patient expresses or implies that he/she is acquiring/has acquired a perceived functionality expectancy set).
2. *Check your work with the criterion answers on p. 142.*

Statement A

"I've learned that I have to speak out when I want something—can't hold back any more."

Statement B

"I've learned that obtaining the DO is pretty much the luck of the draw. I probably got the weekend off in this situation because the sun was out today. I seem to do better on sunny days than on rainy ones."

Statement C

"Other people tune me out when I raise my voice and get angry or start griping about being treated unfairly. When I just say what I want or don't want in a calm way, others listen to me. This was certainly true in this situation. I'm learning that it matters how I act around people. It looks like they react to me differently, depending on what I do and how I do it."

Statement D

"I'm not sure yet about this behavioral consequence thing. I want to believe that it matters what I do, that I can gain control over how my life goes, but I'm not sure yet. It looks like saying clearly what I wanted in the situation helped me get what I wanted. But I'm not convinced yet. We'll see."

Statement E

"I am really sensitive to the effects I have on others now. It really matters what I do. I used to feel that my life was out of control and this situation is a perfect example of when I used to feel this way. Tom, my supervisor, has always been difficult for me to deal with. I never thought he liked me. In the past, I would have withdrawn when he looked like he didn't like what I was saying. I would have ended up depressed and feeling rejected. Yesterday was different. I hung in there over Tom's initial objections, I was clear about what I wanted to accomplish in the project, I made sure he understood my agenda completely, and then I asked for his decision. I got the green light! And not by accident, I might add. Tom finally saw my point, accepted my rationale, knew exactly what I wanted to do, and he finally agreed to it. When I think about it, people have probably never really known what I wanted. I never hung around long enough to make myself clear. My failure has not been their fault, it's been *mine*. I've finally taken control of my life. I'm not helpless anymore. What I do really matters!"

Statement Rankings

I. _____   II. _____   III. _____   IV. _____   V. _____

Check your work with the criterion answers on p. 142.

Criterion Answers for Step 3 Remediation Exercises

I. _E_   II. _C_   III. _A_   IV. _D_   V. _B_

E—Excellent rationale provided for obtaining the DO. Patient is also generalizing the SA learning to other life areas.

C—Good rationale proposed for DO attainment. Patient is also beginning to generalize in-session learning to other life areas.

A—This response represents the early stages of perceived functionality acquisition.

D—Patient wants to believe that it matters what he/she does but is not quite sure yet.

B—The acquisition of perceived functionality has not yet begun. The clinician must continue to administer SA in order to demonstrate the consequences of behavior.

STEP 4: GENERALIZATION AND TRANSFER OF LEARNING

Review

Review the "Therapist Rule for Administering Step 4" in the text (p. 164) and summarized here:

1. Therapist asks patient to pinpoint a specific interpersonal event that is similar to the just completed SA.

Review the "Patient Performance Goal for Step 4" in the text (p. 165) and summarized here:

1. Patient learns to pinpoint specific similar events where the skills learned in SA can be transferred and applied appropriately.

Exercises

1. *Rank order* the following statements, taken from five chronically depressed patients beginning with the *highest quality statement* denoting generalization/transfer of learning and ending with the lowest. The key discriminating variable is how well the patient is able to pinpoint a specific situation (in space and time) and to explain how the new SA learning is applicable.
2. *Check your work with the criterion answers on p. 145*, which should be covered up while you complete the exercise, because the exercise and answers are on facing pages.

Statement A

"Learning to ask directly for what I want applies to a situation I got into last Monday at the office. My boss asked me to spend a week in Atlanta and clean up some company business there. I really wanted the New York project. I talked around the issue, saying that New York would really be nice in the spring. I never really said that I would rather have the New York job over the Atlanta one. I could have gotten the New York job, had I asked for it specifically. Not being clear about what I wanted means I'm going to Atlanta, and my buddy is going to New York. What we did today in the SA applies directly to that conversation. Next time, I'll ask specifically for what I want."

Statement B

"I can't think of any other situation where I could use what I've learned today. This is the first girlfriend I've ever had, so what I learned today about setting my limits concerning what I don't want doesn't apply to any other area or situation in my life."

Statement C

"It's really hard trying to think of other situations where first thinking about my goal before I go to see my boss would be applicable. It might apply to the way I go about settling disagreements with my wife though I'm not completely certain. Maybe thinking through what I wanted, before we got into the heat of an argument trying to settle something, would make a difference. She and I get into a lot of arguments over things we have disagreed about in the past. Had one hot argument last night over something that had happened earlier in the day. I'm not sure, but maybe planning out what I want first would lead to a better outcome with her."

Statement D

"I can think of a number of situations where being assertive would have helped me get what I want. Yep, being assertive is clearly the best strategy."

Statement E

"Learning to talk with my mother in a calm way without yelling at her always leads to a better outcome. Wish I could have done that when I was in high school. It surely would have made a big difference in how we got along. Sometimes I am over at her house, and I yell at her when she criticizes me for wanting to use her car. She gets angry with me and tells me that I can't use it. If I didn't yell and stayed calm and explained why I needed to borrow her car, I would be able to use it more."

Statement Rankings

I. _____   II. _____   III. _____   IV. _____   V. _____

Check your work with the criterion answers on the facing page.

Criterion Answers for Step 4 Remediation Exercises

I. __A__   II. __E__   III. __C__   IV. __D__   V. __B__

A—A response showing excellent transfer of learning. A specific situation is pinpointed, and the explanation of how the new learning would have been applicable is clearly delineated.

E—All the patient needs to do is pinpoint a time *when* this event occurred and the transfer of learning step is complete.

C—The patient is still somewhat uncertain about how to apply what he has learned. He must learn to be more specific when describing how to transfer learning to other problematical events. You might emphasize that the transfer sentence is very important. Chronically depressed patients think and talk in global ways that mitigate DO attainment. Specific thinking and talking must be facilitated in all areas of living. Step 4 provides another opportunity to do this.

D—The patient has yet to learn the importance of specificity. The clinician must assist the individual to think in specific terms when considering how in-session learning can be transferred to other areas of living. Failure to master Step 4 means that the patient cannot yet apply what is learned in the session to problems on the outside.

B—Very primitive response to Step 4. Much work remains to be done to assist the patient in learning how to transfer and generalize the learning taking place in therapy to problem situations on the outside.

FIVE

Using Disciplined Personal Involvement to Modify Patient Behavior

C hronically depressed patients are better served by clinicians who are willing to engage them with *disciplined personal involvement*, a powerful change vehicle. In this chapter you will learn to use your involvement with patients to modify their behavior. Personal involvement must be informed by two sources of information. First, an empirical description of the *interpersonal style of the patient* can be measured by the Impact Message Inventory (IMI) (Kiesler, 1987, 1996) (see the text, Chapter Eight). Once the interpersonal style of the patient is identified by the therapist, he/she can keep in mind the salient interpersonal *pulls/ tugs* of the patient as the therapy progresses. Another way to say the same thing is that the IMI helps practitioners define patients' *interpersonal stimulus value*. The stimulus value of most chronic patients pulls unwary therapists into assuming dominant and/or hostile roles. If dominance and/or hostility characterize(s) the therapist's behavior, then the effectiveness of treatment will be compromised and behavior change is unlikely.

The second source of information that must guide personal involvement is a relevant set of interpersonal *transference hypotheses* (see the text, pp. 90–104). The therapist's proactive use of the transference hypotheses teaches patients to discriminate between the relationship they have with the clinician and the relationship they had/have with destructive significant others. This process of discrimination often transforms destructive interpersonal histories into corrective emotional experiences.

This portion of the training manual is divided into three parts. Part I describes the rationale for using the IMI to identify the clinician's interpersonal role. The practice exercises in Part I show you how to identify the destructive response tendencies that you will face when you treat chronically depressed patients. Avoiding these response tendencies requires a knowledge of the patient's interpersonal style.

In Part II you will learn how to construct transference hypotheses that are then used to modify patient behavior. Before going any further, I encourage you to review Chapters Eight and Five (in this order) in the text. Chapter Eight discusses the use of the IMI, and Chapter Five illustrates how CBASP therapists construct and utilize the transference hypotheses during the session.

Part III introduces the Interpersonal Discrimination Exercise (IDE). The IDE is the procedure that proactively utilizes the transference hypotheses to modify interpersonal behavior.

PART I
The Impact Message Inventory

OVERVIEW

As noted above, the Impact Message Inventory, or IMI, illustrates the interpersonal stimulus value of the patient by graphically depicting the type of covert pulls/tugs (emotional, cognitive, and behavioral) a particular patient will exert. Examine the octant version of the IMI (Kiesler & Schmidt, 1993) shown in Figure 5.* These pulls/tugs create automatic *behavioral action tendencies* in you that you must learn to inhibit. Kiesler (1996) explains:

> The IMI was constructed on the assumption that the interpersonal or evoking style of Person (A) can be validly defined and measured by assessing the covert responses or "impact messages" of Person(s) (B) during interactions with or observations of A. (p. 28)

In CBASP, Person A is the "patient" and Person B is the psychotherapist. Using the IMI to identify the evoking style (stimulus value) of the patient helps disciplined clinicians avoid reacting to patients, either covertly or overtly, in nonproductive ways. I characterize these knee-jerk dominant and/or hostile interpersonal reactions as danger zones or lethal response tendencies that neutralize effective treatment.

Kiesler (1983, 1996) uses the term *complementarity reaction tendencies* to describe the natural behavioral action tendencies that patients evoke in therapists by their covert and overt pulls/tugs. In psychological terms, complementarity is the natural inclination to behave in certain ways toward others, given their specific stimulus value. For example, submissive interpersonal styles (the patient) naturally pull for dominant reactions (the unwary therapist); conversely, dominant interpersonal behavior (the unwary therapist) pulls for submissive behavior (the patient); hostile behavior (the patient) pulls for hostile counteractions (the unwary therapist); while a friendly interpersonal style (the disciplined therapist) inclines others (patients) to reciprocate in a friendly manner.

The most natural complementarity reactions of clinicians who encounter the modal interpersonal behavior of chronic patients (i.e., submission and hostility) are: (1) to do the work of therapy for patients (dominance); and (2) to react to patients' detached or outright hostile behavior (hostility) with concomitant interpersonal withdrawal/disengagement or actual verbal counter-hostility.

Using Kiesler's sample IMI shown in Figure 5 makes it possible for us to illustrate graphically the characterizations of impact identified in Figure 6. You may find that you think of other reaction tendencies as you consider these sentences; remember that Kiesler's descriptive reactions are based on the IMI content items for each one of the octants. Chronic patients usually obtain peak (highest) scores in four octants (McCullough et al., 1994):

---

*Figures 5 and 6 are reproduced by special permission of the publisher, Mind Garden, Inc., 1690 Woodside Road #202, Redwood City, CA 94061: (650) 261-3500: from the *Impact Message Inventory* by Donald J. Kiesler. Copyright 1991 and 1995 by Donald J. Kiesler. All rights reserved. Further reproduction is prohibited without the distributor's written consent.

Profile Summary Sheet
IMPACT MESSAGE INVENTORY: FORM IIA OCTANT VERSION
Donald J. Kiesler and James A. Schmidt

Target Person _____
Respondent _____
Date _____

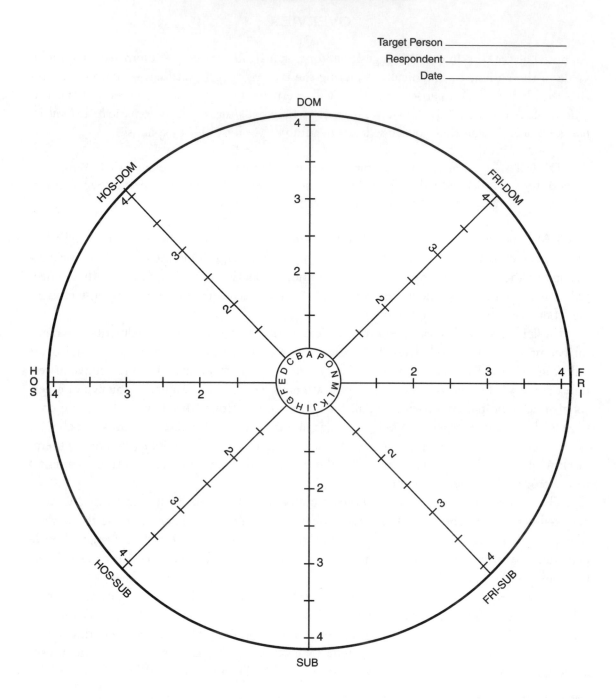

FIGURE 5. Impact Message Inventory completed following session 2. Copyright 1991 by Donald J. Kiesler. All rights reserved.

1. Submissive (helplessness)
2. Hostile-Submissive (anxious/nervous, detached)
3. Hostile (overt attack)
4. Friendly-Submissive (fawning, obsequiousness)

The complementarity reaction tendencies therapists must inhibit when faced with these behaviors are the following:

1. The therapist complementarity pull is for *Dominant* behavior given a patient's peak score in the Submissive Octant, "Do what I say and you'll be okay."
2. The therapist complementarity pull is for *Hostile-Dominant* behavior given a patient's peak score in the Hostile-Submissive Octant, "Your efforts are disappointing; I'll have to do it myself."
3. The therapist complementarity pull is for *Hostile* behavior, given a patient's peak score in the Hostile Octant, "You annoy me, stay away from me."
4. The therapist complementarity pull is for *Friendly-Dominant* behavior, given a patient's peak score in the Friendly-Submissive Octant, "I'm clever and will dazzle you with my talents."

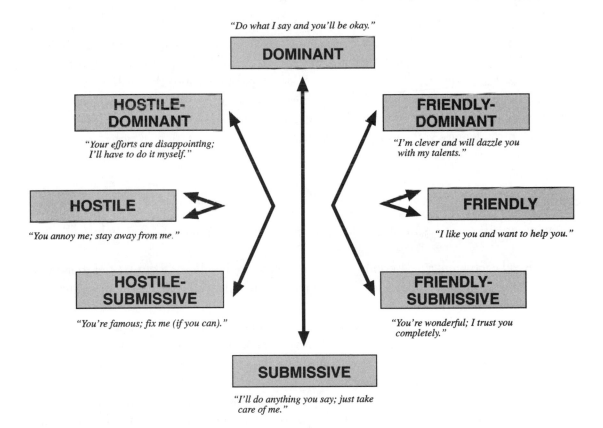

FIGURE 6. Octant Complementary "Pulls" of Kiesler's Interpersonal Circle. Copyright 1995 by Donald J. Kiesler. All rights reserved.

Disciplined personal involvement means that therapists reject the complementarity pulls to be hostile (push away) and dominant (take charge and do the work of therapy for the patient). Instead, CBASP clinicians, using the complementarity information available from the IMI, actualize a disciplined *acomplementarity role* (Kiesler, 1996) that, in effect, says to the individual: "To hell with your attempts to get me to behave like you want. React and deal with me personally in a positive way!" Responding with kindness and encouragement when patients pull for hostility, or reacting with a submissive response ("You do it, I'll wait to see how you manage this task.") when dominance would be the complementary reaction, are examples. Confronting preoperational patients with acomplementarity reactions is similar to the *mismatching demands* of Situational Analysis wherein preoperational patients are required to problem solve using formal operations procedures (see the text, pp. 77, 87–88, 129). When practitioners do not react in complementary ways (which are similar to the way other people typically react to them), patients are automatically thrown into an unfamiliar interpersonal territory that activates, over time, a different (more facilitative) interpersonal level of functioning. The new mismatching experience may produce momentary discomfort because the therapist does not react to the patient in a familiar interpersonal manner; however, acomplementarity reactions offer patients opportunities to learn novel interpersonal patterns.

Administering the IMI Following Session 2

The Impact Message Inventory: Form IIA Octant Scale Version (Kiesler, 1993) can be purchased from its publisher, Mind Garden, Inc., 1690 Woodside Road, Suite 202, Redwood City, CA 94061; (650) 261-3500. CBASP trainees are exposed to the administration and scoring of the IMI at their first CBASP Training Workshop. In addition, they role-play situations wherein they confront the pulls/tugs for dominance and hostility that mimic interactions with chronic patients. We turn now to the Part I exercises that are designed to help you recognize the reaction tendencies you will face when treating the chronic patient. Prior to working the exercises, review the text, Chapter 8.

Exercises

Following are 10 exercises in identifying therapist reaction tendencies. For each:

1. Read each scenario describing what the patient said and/or did during the therapy session. Put yourself in the role of the therapist—the one who is on the *receiving end* of the patient's behavior.

    Note: The *goal* of this exercise is to help you recognize the Kieslerian interpersonal styles of chronic patients and the various complementarity pulls/tugs they exert on you. As you read the scenarios, allow yourself to experience the effects the patient's behavior would have on you (i.e., what the patient's behavior makes you feel/feel like doing/feel like saying), so that the exercises approximate actual in-session impact produced by real patients. *Let yourself experience the pulls/tugs without thinking too much about them—just experience your natural reactions and then rate them by selecting the complementarity octant pull/tug.*

2. Identify the one interpersonal octant that best describes the patient's behavior.

3. Then identify *one* of your "natural" reaction inclinations or tendencies from the four complementarity response choices that follow each scenario. Remember, you are *not* being asked what you would actually do, only what you *naturally feel inclined* to do, given the behavior of the patient. Be as honest with yourself as you can.

   Note: The multiple-choice answers are based on Kiesler's complementarity response tendencies as applied to the interpersonal styles of chronic patients (i.e., Submissive pulls for Dominant; Hostile-Submissive pulls for Hostile-Dominant; Hostile pulls for Hostile; Friendly-Submissive pulls for Friendly-Dominant—see Figure 6).

4. Write out a few sentences that describe how the patient makes you feel.

5. *Check your work with the criterion answers on pp. 159–161.*

Therapist Reaction 1

"Dr. Smith, I have wanted to work with you, and only you. Your reputation is widely known all over the world. I wouldn't want to put my mental well-being in any one else's hands. I'm so glad that you were able to see me. I know that everything is going to be all right. You are just a marvelous doctor."

a. Check the one interpersonal style that best describes this patient:

   1. Submissive ____
   2. Hostile-Submissive ____
   3. Hostile ____
   4. Friendly-Submissive ____

b. Select the one complementarity pull this patient most clearly exerts on you:

   1. "Do what I say and you'll be okay" (Dominant). ____
   2. "Your efforts are disappointing; I'll have to do it myself" (Hostile-Dominant). ____
   3. "You annoy me; stay away from me" (Hostile). ____
   4. "I'm clever and will dazzle you with my talents" (Friendly-Dominant). ____

c. How did the patient make you feel? What did you feel like doing or saying? Be as honest as possible.

   _____

   _____

   _____

Check your work with the criterion answers on p. 159.

Therapist Reaction 2

THERAPIST: I want you to list the persons who have played a significant role in your life. I am talking about individuals who have left their stamp on you, so to speak, who have influenced you to be the kind of person you turned out to be.

PATIENT: I don't want to do this. I don't like this stuff! Nothing can help me. I need to get out of here. You ask me to do things I can't do. I'm just going to fail at this like I fail at everything else. I need to get up and leave. I don't know why I keep sitting here.

a. Check the one interpersonal style that best describes this patient:

   1. Submissive _____
   2. Hostile-Submissive _____
   3. Hostile _____
   4. Friendly-Submissive _____

b. Select the one complementarity pull this patient most clearly exerts on you:

   1. "Do what I say and you'll be okay" (Dominant). _____
   2. "Your efforts are disappointing; I'll have to do it myself" (Hostile-Dominant). _____
   3. "You annoy me; stay away from me" (Hostile). _____
   4. "I'm clever and will dazzle you with my talents" (Friendly-Dominant). _____

c. How did the patient make you feel? What did you feel like doing or saying? Be as honest as possible.

   _____

   _____

   _____

Check your work with the criterion answers on p. 159.

Therapist Reaction 3

"I couldn't do my homework this week. I've thought of little else since our last session. I went home with the intention of telling my husband how he'd hurt me with his mean comments about how I do housework. He keeps telling me that he ought to do it, because I do it wrong. I just couldn't do it. I think the best thing for me to do is to quit coming to see you. All I will do is fail at this therapy, and then you'll hate me the same way my husband does. It's no use. My father told me that I would end up no good—that I couldn't do anything right. He was right. This had better be our last session."

a. Check the one interpersonal style that best describes this patient (remember, withdrawal/detachment is a hostile response):

   1. Submissive _____
   2. Hostile-Submissive _____
   3. Hostile _____
   4. Friendly-Submissive _____

b. Select the one complementarity pull this patient most clearly exerts on you:

   1. "Do what I say and you'll be okay" (Dominant). _____
   2. "Your efforts are disappointing; I'll have to do it myself" (Hostile-Dominant). _____

3. "You annoy me; stay away from me" (Hostile). ____

4. "I'm clever and will dazzle you with my talents" (Friendly-Dominant). ____

c. How did the patient make you feel? What did you feel like doing or saying? Be as honest as possible.

_____

_____

_____

Check your work with the criterion answers on p. 159.

Therapist Reaction 4

"You have asked too much of me. I've never been able to do anything on my own. You are going to have to help me complete my Situational Analysis worksheet. Show me how to do a situational description. What does it mean to do this? Please help me or else I just can't do this stuff."

a. Check the one interpersonal style that best describes this patient:

1. Submissive ____
2. Hostile-Submissive ____
3. Hostile ____
4. Friendly-Submissive ____

b. Select the one complementarity pull this patient most clearly exerts on you:

1. "Do what I say and you'll be okay" (Dominant). ____
2. "Your efforts are disappointing; I'll have to do it myself" (Hostile-Dominant). ____
3. "You annoy me; stay away from me" (Hostile). ____
4. "I'm clever and will dazzle you with my talents" (Friendly-Dominant). ____

c. How did the patient make you feel? What did you feel like doing or saying? Be as honest as possible.

_____

_____

_____

Check your work with the criterion answers on pp. 159–160.

Therapist Reaction 5

"Doc, I don't like getting involved with people. You talked about me not trusting you. You're right. I don't trust you and I'm not going to let myself trust you. I got burned once by putting all my eggs in one basket with someone. It will never happen again—certainly not here."

a. Check the one interpersonal style that best describes this patient:

   1. Submissive ____
   2. Hostile-Submissive ____
   3. Hostile ____
   4. Friendly-Submissive ____

b. Select the one complementarity pull this patient most clearly exerts on you:

   1. "Do what I say and you'll be okay" (Dominant). ____
   2. "Your efforts are disappointing; I'll have to do it myself" (Hostile-Dominant). ____
   3. "You annoy me; stay away from me" (Hostile). ____
   4. "I'm clever and will dazzle you with my talents" (Friendly-Dominant). ____

c. How did the patient make you feel? What did you feel like doing or saying? Be as honest as possible.

   _____

   _____

   _____

Check your work with the criterion answers on p. 160.

Therapist Reaction 6

Therapist's notes: The patient complains frequently and passionately about the negative way her husband treats her. She says that he hurts her by what he says, she calls him "emotionally insensitive," and she provides numerous examples of how he won't talk to her when she tries to share her feelings. Often, she will give examples of how he gets mad at her whenever she makes the slightest mistake. She describes him as "overreacting" about every mistake she makes. Whenever I try to focus on her behavior and what she did prior to the husband's negative reaction, she begins to cry, saying that she fails at everything and can't do anything right; she becomes nervous and fidgety and complains that I always take the husband's side, and that he never sees things her way or tries to help her. Attempts to identify her antecedent behavior that provokes the husband's response is always blocked by a withdrawal into crying, self-chastisement, or outright refusal to discuss her behavior.

a. Check the interpersonal style that best describes this patient:

   1. Submissive ____
   2. Hostile-Submissive ____
   3. Hostile ____
   4. Friendly-Submissive ____

b. Select the one complementarity pull this patient most clearly exerts on you:

   1. "Do what I say and you'll be okay" (Dominant). ____
   2. "Your efforts are disappointing; I'll have to do it myself" (Hostile-Dominant). ____

3. "You annoy me; stay away from me" (Hostile). _____
4. "I'm clever and will dazzle you with my talents (Friendly-Dominant). _____

c. How did the patient make you feel? What did you feel like doing or saying? Be as honest as possible.

_____

_____

_____

Check your work with the criterion answers on p. 160.

Therapist Reaction 7

"Dr. Hardy, when you explain things to me, I see them so clearly. I don't know why my other therapists didn't explain things the way you do. I understand now why I've been depressed. I trusted you from the time I first met you. There's just something about the way you talk that makes me know that I'm listening to the truth. I'll do anything you say, just keep telling me how to beat this depression. I think you are a wonderful therapist."

a. Check the interpersonal style that best describes this patient:

1. Submissive _____
2. Hostile-Submissive _____
3. Hostile _____
4. Friendly-Submissive _____

b. Select the one complementarity pull this patient most clearly exerts on you:

1. "Do what I say and you'll be okay" (Dominant). _____
2. "Your efforts are disappointing; I'll have to do it myself" (Hostile-Dominant). _____
3. "You annoy me; stay away from me" (Hostile). _____
4. "I'm clever and will dazzle you with my talents" (Friendly-Dominant). _____

c. How did this patient make you feel? What did you feel like doing or saying? Be as honest as possible.

_____

_____

_____

Check your work with the criterion answers on p. 160.

Therapist Reaction 8

PATIENT: Doc, I really become nervous whenever you focus on me and ask me questions about why I do things. I feel exposed, and I don't like people to know me this well.

THERAPIST: Can you give me an example of *when* you felt this way.

PATIENT: Sure—last week when we did that Situational Analysis on the disagreement my boss and I had. I had to concentrate on what the situation meant to me, and on what I said and how I said it. I got so nervous I couldn't think straight. I don't like talking about myself around you or anyone else. Any time I've done this in the past, I've just clammed up, gotten quiet, and not said anything more.

THERAPIST: Where does your nervousness about disclosure come from?

PATIENT: My parents always punished me when I told them what I had done. I was usually wrong, I admit, but I learned early that I had to cover my tracks and either lie or say nothing. I can't do these SAs. You and I need to do another kind of therapy. This CBASP therapy is not going to work for me. I just can't talk about myself this way. It's too scary for me.

a. Check the one interpersonal style that best describes this patient:

    1. Submissive _____
    2. Hostile-Submissive _____
    3. Hostile _____
    4. Friendly-Submissive _____

b. Select the one complementarity pull this patient most clearly exerts on you:

    1. "Do what I say and you'll be okay" (Dominant). _____
    2. "Your efforts are disappointing; I'll have to do it myself" (Hostile-Dominant). _____
    3. "You annoy me; stay away from me" (Hostile). _____
    4. "I'm clever and will dazzle you with my talents" (Friendly-Dominant). _____

c. How did the patient make you feel? What did you feel like doing or saying? Be as honest as possible.

_____

_____

_____

Check your work with the criterion answers on pp. 160–161.

Therapist Reaction 9

THERAPIST: What do you do to get to know the patients on your unit?

PATIENT: I just read their charts.

THERAPIST: I mean, what do you do to build a relationship with them?

PATIENT: As little as possible. I spend a lot of time in the nurses' station. I talk to them if they are being quiet—but only for a short period of time.

a. Check the interpersonal style that best describes this patient:

  1. Submissive ____
  2. Hostile-Submissive ____
  3. Hostile ____
  4. Friendly-Submissive ____

b. Select the one complementarity pull this patient most clearly exerts on you:

  1. "Do what I say and you'll be okay" (Dominant). ____
  2. "Your efforts are disappointing; I'll have to do it myself" (Hostile-Dominant). ____
  3. "You annoy me; stay away from me" (Hostile). ____
  4. "I'm clever and will dazzle you with my talents" (Friendly-Dominant). ____

c. How did this patient make you feel? What did you feel like doing or saying? Be as honest as possible.

  _____

  _____

  _____

Check your work with the criterion answers on p. 161.

Therapist Reaction 10

Therapist's notes: The patient comes to the first therapy session looking detached, very nervous, and takes a seat. She didn't speak to me or make any sort of eye contact. Both hands lay open in her lap in a supplicating manner, with the palms upward. The patient keeps looking at the floor or at the wall. When I asked why she has come for therapy, she replied in a quiet, almost inaudible way that she has been depressed. She does not speak voluntarily, only if I ask a question, and then the replies are made in an almost painful manner. When the hour is completed, I notice that she looks nervous, tired, and exhausted. An appointment is made for another session the following week. I am not looking forward to another hour of such hard work.

a. Check the one interpersonal style that best describes this patient:

  1. Submissive ____
  2. Hostile-Submissive ____
  3. Hostile ____
  4. Friendly-Submissive ____

b. Select the one complementarity pull this patient most clearly exerts on you:

  1. "Do what I say and you'll be okay" (Dominant). ____
  2. "Your efforts are disappointing; I'll have to do it myself" (Hostile-Dominant). ____

3. "You annoy me; stay away from me" (Hostile). ____

4. "I'm clever and will dazzle you with my talents" (Friendly-Dominant). ____

c. How did this patient make you feel? What did you feel like doing or saying? Be as honest as possible.

_____

_____

_____

Check your work with the criterion answers on p. 161.

Criterion Answers for Part I Exercises

Therapist Reaction 1

 a. Friendly-Submissive.
 b. Friendly-Dominant.
 c. Such patients are flattering and fawning in the way they relate to psychotherapists. The task of therapy is to refuse to provide the complementarity response of becoming over-confident in the face of the excessive flattery (Friendly-Dominant) and to remain task-oriented. Helping the patient become more independent and assertive is the goal (i.e., to "even things up" interpersonally whereby the therapist is perceived in a more realistic manner).

Therapist Reaction 2

 a. Hostile.
 b. Hostile.
 c. This is the type of patient who comes in swinging, and the blows land squarely on the jaw of the therapist. The knee-jerk pull/tug on most clinicians is to feel, think, or want to say: "Screw you! If you don't want to work with me, then get out of my office!" Countering hostility with hostility is the reflexive complementarity response. Since this reaction is counter-productive, CBASP therapists learn other ways to react. (To manage this type of assault, for starters, read the text, pp. 177–183.)

Therapist Reaction 3

 a. Hostile-Submissive.
 b. Hostile-Dominant.
 c. If your reaction went something like this—"Damn, you'll never get it together! I thought we had worked all this out last week. Maybe if I went home with you and held your hand you could stand up to your old man!"—then your reaction is similar to mine! Skinner (1956) said that if the organism doesn't behave the way we want, then we've asked too much, too quickly; organisms "always behave as they ought" (Skinner, 1956, p. 233). Inhibiting the Hostile-Dominant complementarity reaction in this instance is necessary. The patient is not yet ready to change her behavior.

Therapist Reaction 4

 a. Submissive.
 b. Dominant.
 c. The pull/tug here is for the therapist to take over, assume a dominant role (the complementarity reaction), and to do the work for the patient. Structure your sessions so that patients must do all the work. Enforcing this criterion is laborious, time-consuming, and often frustrating. But don't do it any other way! Ask yourself this: "What is the

complementarity response for my dominance?" You've got it—*submission*! Maintaining submissiveness is not the psychotherapy goal for the chronic patient!

Therapist Reaction 5

a. Hostile.

b. Hostile.

c. Listening to an individual like this makes one want to say, "Get out of my presence! You wear me out with your griping." As discussed earlier, returning hostility with hostility is the complementarity response, and it is always counterproductive. The therapist can rest assured that he/she is the brunt of this man's remarks when he discusses his psychotherapy with others. Short-circuiting these in-session global tirades with specific SA work and using the Interpersonal Discrimination Exercise to open up alternative paths for interpersonal interactions is a better way to proceed.

Therapist Reaction 6

a. Hostile-Submissive.

b. Hostile-Dominant.

c. Therapists become frustrated when patients repeatedly avoid problematical situations. The reflexive pull/tug here is the following response tendency: "Dammit to hell! Quit crying and bellyaching and let's deal with the problem!" This is the complementarity Hostile-Dominant reaction. Your frustration is normal and predictable. Learning to inhibit these reaction tendencies is worth the effort. The key here is to continue to focus the patient on SA work and to allow the SA method to demonstrate to the patient that her behavior with the husband is maintaining the problem.

Therapist Reaction 7

a. Friendly-Submissive.

b. Friendly-Dominant.

c. Did you feel warm and flattered inside, and then did you want to impress the patient even more? If you did, you reacted in a quite normal way. You must inhibit this reaction tendency, though, and keep focusing the patient on the consequences of her behavior. One consequence of her Friendly-Submissive style is that she overlooks her own strengths as long as she stays focused on the strengths of others. Accentuating the former and modifying the latter is the goal here.

Therapist Reaction 8

a. Hostile-Submissive.

b. Hostile-Dominant.

c. The patient is mildly pleading with the therapist to remove him from the "hotseat." It's obvious that he is uncomfortable with the SA method because he fears having to divulge his failures in the presence of the clinician. The complementarity response goes something like this: "Oh, come on, this isn't so bad. You're not going to die by focusing on these issues!" This is *not* the tact to take. Again, continuing to concentrate on the behavioral consequences in SA should reduce the anxiety over time. Use the Interpersonal Discrimination Exercise to demonstrate that the therapist's reactions to his difficulties/mistakes are quite different when compared to his parents'. This patient's discomfort will not be resolved quickly; it will definitely take time.

Therapist Reaction 9

a. Hostile.
b. Hostile.
c. The complementarity response would be the following: "Good grief! Why did I ever come to work today? This idiot is going to be a pain in the ass. I feel like I've got to trot out all my professional credentials. I wish he'd get lost!" The hostile patient is difficult for all of us. Anger pushes everyone away and keeps others at a distance. The goal of treatment is not responding in kind. Rather, it is to help this individual learn to relate to a person (the clinician) who refuses to allow himself/herself to be pushed away.

Therapist Reaction 10

a. Hostile-Submissive.
b. Hostile-Dominant.
c. Many of our scenarios in Part I have dealt with Hostile-Submissive patients. This is because they fill up our offices. Avoiding the Hostile-Dominant response tendency is achieved by demonstrating to this woman the effects of her behavior. Unknowingly, she is driving people away by behaving in a Hostile-Submissive manner. SA will illustrate this fact and so will the Interpersonal Discrimination Exercise (IDE). In addition, the IDE will help her discriminate between the positive behavior of the therapist and the negative behavior of significant others. Thus will she come to see the inappropriateness of her Hostile-Submissive behavior with the clinician. SA will demonstrate how she cannot achieve her DOs using this response style.

Steps Leading to the Construction
of the Transference Hypotheses

Section A
DERIVING THE CAUSAL THEORY CONCLUSIONS

Part I helped you see that being aware of the interpersonal stimulus value of chronic patients sensitizes you to their strong pulls/tugs for dominance and hostility. Once these complementarity response tendencies are inhibited, disciplined personal involvement can be effectively administered to modify the patient's behavior. The technique used for this purpose is the Interpersonal Discrimination Exercise (IDE). The IDE highlights interpersonal behavioral consequences, teaches formal operations thinking, and enhances motivation for change. Using the IDE, you will learn to (1) obtain a "significant other history," (2) deduce "causal theory conclusions" from this history, and (3) construct one or more transference hypotheses. You will also gain practice in conducting the steps leading to transference hypothesis formulation.

Transference, or the learned patterns of behavior which patients enact with people (including the therapist), is an important concern for the CBASP therapist. Most chronically depressed patients easily recall developmental histories that include trauma. They frequently transfer negative interpersonal expectancies as well as overt behaviors that accrue from their developmental histories to the therapeutic relationship. Proactively modifying the negative transference, which functions as an interpersonal obstacle, is often necessary if treatment is to be successful. If the negative transference problems are not corrected and replaced by more appropriate interpersonal expectancies and behavior, these problems will sabotage the therapist-patient relationship and preclude change. Modification of these learned negative interpersonal expectancies and behaviors is the goal of the IDE.

Introduction to Session 2

Session 2 is spent obtaining a significant other history. During the history intake, patients are asked to formulate *causal hypotheses* about how growing up around each significant other has influenced the direction their lives have taken. Asking patients to make causal connections between the behavior of significant others and its effects is a mismatching exercise requiring formal operational thinking. The request is made to these preoperational patients for two reasons: to help them begin to think causally about their lives (in an "if this . . . then that" manner) and to obtain whatever causal information patients can generate so that the transference hypotheses will be relevant.

Following the completion of session 2, the clinician utilizes the recalled historical material as well as the patient's causal conclusions about each person on the list and deduces causal theory conclusions about each significant other.

Let's take a case example of a male patient (seen by a female practitioner) who described his mother as the type of person who punished him in a ridiculing manner for showing any emotion. When questioned about how growing up around his mother had influenced the direction his life had taken (causal thinking), he replied that because of her he has always been reticent to let anyone, particularly women, know how he feels. The causal theory conclusion the therapist drew from the history on the mother was as follows:

> *Causal theory conclusion concerning mother:* "When I am around others, particularly women, I cannot express how I feel. I always clam up and keep my feelings to myself."

One or two transference hypotheses are then constructed (see the text, Table 5.1, p. 94, for an example of how this procedure is conducted) based on the salient interpersonal themes available from the several causal theory conclusions.

I will digress for a moment and reiterate the four transference hypotheses domains to which the causal theory conclusions must be connected. Remember, each hypothesis describes specifically what the patient believes will happen to him/her while with the therapist. The hypothesis for the *intimacy/closeness* domain has already been mentioned in the example above. Next are situations in which the patient expresses/discloses a *particular emotional need/problem* to the clinician, either verbally or nonverbally. For example, one patient with an incestuous history with her father frequently sexualized all aspects of the therapeutic relationship. She often made suggestive overtures when she was fearful, lonely, or undecided/confused about something. The male clinician identified these emotional needs and, by not replicating the father's behavior, helped the woman discriminate her fear, loneliness, and confused emotional needs from sexual arousal. Then he taught his patient to behave in a different way, based on the particular felt need. For example, if she was fearful or lonely, she told the clinician; if she was undecided or confused about something, she learned to label the baffling experience and connect it to the problem at hand.

Another interpersonal domain covered by a transference hypothesis involves *failing* or *making mistakes* around the clinician. Early-onset patients regularly present a developmental history wherein failure was severely punished or ridiculed. When this theme is salient, a transference hypothesis is then formulated and, using the IDE, the practitioner helps the patient cope with a perceived failure by discriminating between the accepting behavior of the therapist and the negative reactions of significant others.

The final interpersonal transference domain involves encounters in which patients experience and/or act out (verbally or nonverbally) *negative affect* toward the therapist. These emotions may include fear, frustration, anger, shame, guilt, disappointment, and so on. Again, patients will have described a significant other history in which expressing negative affect resulted in interpersonal rejection or outright punishment. A transference hypothesis is then constructed to cover occasions when negative affect is experience and/or expressed. Again, remember that the transference hypothesis refers specifically to what the patient (implicitly or explicitly) believes will happen to him/her while with the therapist.

Returning to the case example above, let's see how the therapist constructed one of the transference hypotheses.

The causal theory conclusion about the mother influenced the way the therapist constructed the *closeness/intimacy* transference hypothesis. The hypothesis would apply to any type of *closeness/intimacy* interpersonal experience the pair might encounter. As noted above, the transference hypotheses are always stated in an "if this . . . then that" format, with the name of the clinician inserted (the therapist is the protagonist in the hypothesis sentence). The female therapist constructed the following hypothesis:

> "*If* I let Dr. Samuel know how I feel (about anything), *then* she will punish/ridicule me" (Closeness/intimacy).

Once the hypothesis is formulated, it can be used proactively in the IDE to help the patient discriminate between the destructive consequences delivered by the mother following emotional disclosure and the positive consequences administered by Dr. Samuel for similar behavior.

A final caveat about transference hypothesis construction must be made. Limit yourself to no more than one or two transference hypotheses per patient. One or two will be sufficient and will allow you adequate time to address both the interpersonal expectancies and the behaviors. The rule of thumb for hypothesis construction is this:

> *Rule*: Be parsimonious. Construct hypotheses for only the most prominent interpersonal issues! If it appears that more than two are justified, pick the two most salient problem areas and cover these thoroughly during therapy.

Review

Review the steps for eliciting the significant other history in the text (pp. 87–90) and summarized here:

1. Ask the patient to think back over his/her life and list the persons who have been the major players/significant others. Emphasize that we are not talking about listing individuals who are merely acquaintances or friends, but rather persons who have influenced the patient to be the kind of person they have turned out to be.
2. Stress that these life-influencing significant others may have played *either* a positive or negative role.
3. Write down the list in the order the patient provides.
4. When the list is complete, review it in the order provided by the patient. (*Don't* rearrange the order based on your conjecture of who you think may be most important, next most important, etc.).
5. Going down the list, ask the patient to tell you *how* each significant other has left their stamp on him/her; that is, to explain to you *how* the person has influenced the "direction" one's life has taken. *Note*: This is a causal theory request asking the patient to link the behavior of the significant other with its effects on the patient's life.
6. *Do not* suggest causal linkages to the patient. Let the patient do the work without assistance. If the patient cannot construct the causal linkage, move on to the next person

on the list and try again. Most patients will be able to make at least rudimentary hook-ups between the significant other's behavior and its effects.

7. Avoid letting patients ramble on, in a stream-of-consciousness fashion, recounting events that happened with a significant other. Such information does not lead to "if this . . . then that" causal theory conclusions.

8. If a patient provides a list of greater than seven names (some obsessive individuals often do), stop the history-taking after the seventh name.

9. If basic significant other persons are left off the list (e.g., mother, father, siblings), an inquiry should be made as to the reason for the omissions. If one or both parents have been omitted, history and causal theory information should be obtained on these individuals.

Review the goal for the significant other history in the text (p. 88) and summarized here:

1. Patient makes causal connections between the behavior of significant others and their effects on his/her life.

   Note: Some preoperational patients will be unable to make these connections. When this occurs, the therapist must formulate the causal theory conclusions and transference hypotheses with less corroborating information.

Exercises

Following are six exercises for identifying therapist errors. For each:

1. Review each therapist prompt for the significant other history procedure.
2. Using the therapist guidelines listed above, identify the prompt mistake and write it down in the space provided.
3. *Check your work with the criterion answers on p. 168.*

Therapist Errors 1

"Give me the names of persons you are close to and I'll list them."

Pinpoint the mistake(s) and write it out: _____

_____

_____

Check your work with the criterion answers on p. 168.

Therapist Errors 2

"You've given me a list of 13 names. Let's go through the list, and I'll ask you something about each person."

Pinpoint the mistake(s) and write it out: _____

_____

_____

Check your work with the criterion answers on p. 168.

Therapist Errors 3

"You've given me a list of six significant others: mother, father, your brother Philip, your maternal grandmother, your girlfriend Shirley, and your husband Bill. Let's start with Bill first. Tell me how Bill has influenced you to be the kind of person you are."

Pinpoint the mistake(s) and write it out: _____

_____

_____

Check your work with the criterion answers on p. 168.

Therapist Errors 4

"Let's go back through your list, taking each person individually. Tell me what kinds of things you did as a child with the first significant other you listed—that would be your mother."

Pinpoint the mistake(s) and write it out: _____

_____

_____

Check your work with the criterion answers on p. 168.

Therapist Errors 5

"You listed your mother first and said that she was on your case about everything you ever did. You also said she still is. Do you think this might be why you have had so much difficulty with the women you're dating?"

Pinpoint the mistake(s) and write it out: _____

_____

_____

Check your work with the criterion answers on p. 168.

Therapist Errors 6

"You have given me a significant other list of six names: Your father, mother, your sister Theresa, your fourth-grade teacher Mr. Harrington, your paternal grandmother MaMa, and your uncle Bob. Let's go through your list one by one, and see if we can pinpoint how each one has left his/her personal stamp on you. As you talk about each person on the list, try to help me understand how that individual influenced you to be the kind of person you turned out to be. I'm going to take some notes as you talk about each one. Let's start first with your father. How did he influence you to be the kind of person you turned out to be?"

Pinpoint the mistake(s) and write it out: _____

_____

_____

Check your work with the criterion answers on p. 168.

Criterion Answers for Part II, Section A, Exercises

Therapist Errors 1

1. No request for life review of significant others is made.
2. Significant persons not specified nor definition of significant others offered to the patient.
3. No effort is made to list persons who have had a positive or negative influence on the patient.

Therapist Errors 2

1. Too many names have been listed.
2. No effort is made to explain that the goal of the exercise is to identify the type of influence (positive or negative) each significant other has had on the patient.

Therapist Errors 3

1. Therapist has *rearranged* the order of the patient's list.

Therapist Errors 4

1. Therapist has given an *inappropriate prompt* to obtain history information about the mother. The goal here is to determine the mother's influence on the patient, not to delineate the things the patient did with the mother.

Therapist Errors 5

1. Therapist starts out right in determining that the patient's mother is "still on his case about everything."
2. However, he/she makes a mistake by proposing a causal theory conclusion to the patient. Let the patient make the causal connection.

Therapist Errors 6

1. This prompt is a criterion-level performance.

Section B
DEDUCING THE CAUSAL THEORY CONCLUSIONS

Review

Review the material on deducing the causal theory conclusions in the text (pp. 91–95) and summarized here:

1. Summarize the patient's causal inferences about each significant other (*correct prompt*: "What was it like growing up around this person and how did this individual influence the direction your life has taken?" or "What was 'the stamp' this person left on your life?") in a one-sentence statement.
2. The statement should causally link (in an hypothesis manner) the significant other's behavior with the patient's current behavior or generalized expectancies.

Examples

"My father sexually molested me; *therefore*, I expect males to try to use me."

"My mother never loved me; *therefore*, no one could love or care for me."

"My father never did anything but tell me I was "a failure, a loser"; *therefore*, I expect all male authority figures to react the same way."

"Every time I asked my father to help me, he laughed at me and told me: 'Son, real men don't need help from others.' *Therefore*, I never ask for what I need."

"My mother punished me [male patient] every time I made a mistake or messed up; *therefore*, I either hide my mistakes from others or run away from people [quit a job, never ask a woman out twice, etc.] when I make an error."

"When I reached puberty and started developing breasts and looking like a woman, my father rarely spoke to me; *therefore*, men don't care about women, all they want is sex."

Exercises

Following are five causal theory conclusion exercises. For each:

1. Review each scenario (taken from therapists' notes) concerning the influence(s) the significant other(s) had on the patient.
2. Deduce a one-sentence conclusion from the scenario that summarizes the causal influence(s).

Example: If a male patient recalls numerous examples in the significant other history in which his father punished him for making mistakes, then the deduced causal theory conclusion would go something like this: "If I make a mistake, I will be punished." If the "punishment for making mistakes" theme emerges in the significant other history as a prominent motif in the patient's life, then this theme will make a viable candidate for the "making a mistake around the therapist" transference hypothesis (especially if the therapist is male).

3. Indicate the "best-fit" transference hypothesis domain for each causal theory conclusion: intimacy/closeness; emotional needs/problems; failure or making mistakes; negative affect felt/expressed toward the therapist.
4. *Check your work with the criterion answers on p. 173.*

Causal Conclusion 1

SIGNIFICANT OTHER HISTORY: MOTHER

"She drank a lot and when she got mad, which was most of the time, she used to punish me and my sister with a belt. I carried whelps around on my back and legs for days after one of those whippings. I got beatings for everything I did wrong. If I even left one of my dinner dishes on the table and didn't put it in the sink, I got beat. Even today at work or when I'm with my wife, if I make a mistake or mess up—even on something small—my stomach ties up in knots. That's ridiculous, isn't it?"

a. Causal theory conclusion: _____

_____

_____

b. "Best-fit" transference hypothesis domain: _____

_____

Check your work with the criterion answers on p. 173.

Causal Conclusion 2

SIGNIFICANT OTHER HISTORY: FATHER

"He drank all the time. When he got drunk, he would come into my bedroom and get into my bed. I used to pretend I was asleep. He would feel my breasts and then he would put his finger in my vagina. I could hear his heavy breathing and smell the alcohol. I used to play like I was someone else or someplace else. Got to where I wouldn't feel a thing he did to me. He would make himself ejaculate on me, and then he'd leave. I've never had a good relationship with a man. When I start to like a guy, I start getting nervous and finally refuse to go out with him. Guys really don't understand me at all."

a. Causal theory conclusion: _____

_____

_____

b. "Best-fit" transference hypothesis domain: _____

_____

Check your work with the criterion answers on p. 173.

Causal Conclusion 3

SIGNIFICANT OTHER HISTORY: MOTHER

"Mother was never around when we were growing up. I can remember coming home from school, and she was never there. I often fixed supper for my two brothers. No one else did it. Guess I played the 'mother' for my brothers. When she was around, she rarely spoke to me. I remember when I went to her to ask her how to do something—say, run the washing machine—she would always say, 'Ask me another time.' I really don't know who she was or is. I would never go to her if I needed anything, or for advice or help. In fact, I don't go to anyone if I need anything. Guess I'm really like her in that regard. I don't want to be like her, but I am!"

a. Causal theory conclusion: _____
_____
_____

b. "Best-fit" transference hypothesis domain: _____
_____

Check your work with the criterion answers on p. 173.

Causal Conclusion 4

SIGNIFICANT OTHER HISTORY: OLDER BROTHER

"He was outstanding in everything he tried. He made straight A's in school, he was all-district in basketball and track, he got into a first-rate college because of his SAT scores, and he made good grades at college. He is a successful businessman today. God, I gave up competing with him in high school. I just never measured up. People kept expecting me to be like him—my parents, teachers, coaches, everyone. I learned that I will always disappoint others, and they will end up disgusted with me. You will end up that way, too, just wait and see. You'll end up disappointed in me. I just can't win with anyone who really gets to know me. I'm a born loser."

a. Causal theory conclusion: _____
_____
_____

b. "Best-fit" transference hypothesis domain: _____
_____

Check your work with the criterion answers on p. 173.

Causal Conclusion 5

SIGNIFICANT OTHER HISTORY: FATHER

"My father was a marine drill instructor at Quantico. He retired after 20 years in late 1995. He's been a security guard at a trucking firm ever since he left the service. I pity anyone who crosses him after hours. Dad demanded that I do everything in a respectful way. I always had to say, 'Yes sir—No sir' to him. Everything was *sir*. Once I got angry with him and told him that he made me mad because he was unfair and unreasonable. I was grounded for a week for my 'insubordination.' He never wanted to hear about my anger or any other negative feelings. I was taught to behave like the 'son of a marine.' If I didn't like something or someone, I was taught to shut up and do my duty. I've always been that way."

a. Causal theory conclusion: _____

_____

_____

b. "Best-fit" transference hypothesis domain: _____

_____

Check your work with the criterion answers on p. 173.

Criterion Answers for Part II, Section B, Exercises

Causal Conclusion 1

1. With my mother: "I expect to be severely punished for any mistake I make."
2. Failure or making mistakes in front of the therapist.

Causal Conclusion 2

1. With my father: "Getting close to a man means that I will be sexually violated or hurt."
2. Intimacy/closeness with the therapist.

Causal Conclusion 3

1. With my mother: "I can never get anything I need from others."
2. Felt emotional needs/problems in relation to the therapist.

Causal Conclusion 4

1. With my older brother: "I will never measure up; I screw up around people who really get to know me—I'm a born loser."
2. Intimacy/closeness with the therapist.

Causal Conclusion 5

1. With my father: "I cannot express any negative feelings to anyone—I must stay positive and do my duty."
2. Negative affect felt/expressed toward the therapist.

Section C
CONSTRUCTING THE TRANSFERENCE HYPOTHESES

Review

Review the material on constructing the transference hypotheses in the text (pp. 90–98) and summarized here:

1. When you complete the significant other history exercise, review your causal theory conclusions and construct one or two transference hypotheses that represent the most serious interpersonal issues/problems.
2. The "if this . . . then that" format of the transference hypothesis does two things: (a) it names the antecedent problem behavior/situation (*if this* happens); and (b) it describes the expected negative consequence (based on the causal theory conclusion) (. . . *then that* will occur). The therapist names himself/herself as the deliverer of the hurtful consequences.
3. Examples of the four domains for transference hypothesis construction are the following:

   a. "If I get *close* to Dr. Smith, then she will reject me (Intimacy/closeness)."
   b. "If I need to ask Dr. Gannon for *emotional support* to deal with my spouse, then he will not want to provide it" (Emotional need).
   c. "If I *fail* or *make a mistake* around Dr. Holcombe, then he will ridicule me and make me feel like an imbecile" (Failure/mistakes).
   d. "If I *become angry* with Dr. Sylvia and *let him know how I feel*, then he will reject me and tell me not to come back" (Negative affect).

Exercises

Following are four transference hypothesis exercises. For each:

1. Note the gender of the patient and therapist in each exercise.
2. Review the causal theory conclusions extracted from the significant other history material.
3. Select the most serious interpersonal issue/problem and construct *one* "if this . . . then that" transference hypothesis.
4. Use the name of the therapist as the deliverer of the hurtful consequences.
5. Label the implicated transference domain.
6. *Check your work with the criterion answers on p. 178.*

Transference Hypothesis 1

Participants: Female patient; female therapist, Dr. Davis

CAUSAL THEORY CONCLUSION: MOTHER

"Making a mistake around my mother led to my being locked out of the house; therefore, I try extra hard not to make any mistakes. When I make them, I always wait for the hammer to fall. I try to be perfect in everything I do. That way I can avoid making mistakes."

CAUSAL THEORY CONCLUSION: FATHER

"My dad never used to do anything with me. In fact, he spent little time with me because he was always working. I don't expect guys to take much of an interest in me. They don't seem to."

CAUSAL THEORY CONCLUSION: OLDER SISTER

"Betty teased me a lot, and there was a lot of competition between us. We still compete whenever we're around each other. I think I'm very competitive with most women I meet."

a. Construct a transference hypothesis that designates the most serious interpersonal problem:

_____

_____

_____

b. Identify the implicated transference domain: _____

Check your work with the criterion answers on p. 178.

Transference Hypothesis 2

Participants: Male patient; male therapist, Dr. Hays

CAUSAL THEORY CONCLUSION: FATHER

"My dad was a tough guy to get to know. I don't think I ever really knew him. But I really knew his anger. He would get mad at me at the drop of a hat. What I learned was to keep my distance from him. Trying to get close always led to him getting mad at me for doing something wrong. I just learned to keep my distance. I think that I am generally uneasy getting close to others. Others really don't know me, and I don't do much to help them out."

CAUSAL THEORY CONCLUSION: MOTHER

"My mother was a flurry of activity. She was always busy and doing several things at one time. She was not a very affectionate person, and I don't remember ever seeing my mother and father embrace, kiss, or express any physical affection toward each other. I guess they loved each other, at least they said they did. Getting close to others has always been a perplexing thing to me. Not really sure I know how."

CAUSAL THEORY CONCLUSION: UNCLE

"He was a fun guy to be around. He seemed so easy going. During the Second World War, he sent me a metal bracelet made out of the wing of a Japanese plane, a Zero, I think. After the war, he stayed in touch with me, and we used to fish together. He died some years ago, and I really miss him. Good things with guys don't last. It doesn't do much good to get close."

CAUSAL THEORY CONCLUSION: HIGH SCHOOL TEACHER

"I was very close to a teacher in high school. I used to visit her room during lunch periods, and we'd talk. She was a real friend to me. Don't know what happened to us during my senior year. We got together less and less, and then I didn't see her again. She died a few years ago. I just have never counted on a good relationship lasting."

a. Construct a transference hypothesis that designates the most serious interpersonal problem:

_____

_____

_____

b. Identify the implicated transference domain: _____

Check your work with the criterion answers on p. 178.

Transference Hypothesis 3

Participants: Male patient; female therapist, Dr. Smith

CAUSAL THEORY CONCLUSION: MOTHER

"The thing that was most important to her was how things looked to others. She was always talking about doing the right thing so people would like you. It mattered to her how I dressed, because she said that dressing well made people really like you. I could never just relax and be casual—I might do something wrong and others wouldn't like it. I was always taught to be on my best behavior. If I made a mistake, I had to hide it so others wouldn't know I had done anything wrong. Looking good, not screwing up, was the order of the day. I'm still like this—very sensitive about what I do for fear that I will make a mistake and have someone think badly of me."

CAUSAL THEORY CONCLUSION: FATHER

"My father was just the opposite of my mother. He was sloppy and didn't care what other people thought. They always argued about what he did, how he dressed. She never seemed satisfied with him, and she seemed to be embarrassed to be with him in public. I'll never know why they ever married. They were opposites in every way. I could never be sloppy like my dad. My mother was on my case too much. I've always felt that women don't like guys very much."

CAUSAL THEORY CONCLUSION: YOUNGER SISTER

"We were close when we were in elementary school. She is one year younger than I am. After I got to high school, we sort of went our separate ways. She married an airline pilot and has two kids and seems to be doing okay. I like to think that we are close, but I don't see her very often. I really don't know how she feels about me—it's probably not good."

a. Construct a transference hypothesis that designates the most serious interpersonal problem:

_____

_____

_____

b. Identify the implicated transference domain: _____

Check your work with the criterion answers on p. 178.

Transference Hypothesis 4

Participants: Female patient; male therapist, Dr. Emory

CAUSAL THEORY CONCLUSION: FATHER

"He was an alcoholic. Looking back on my childhood, I always had to take care of him. He couldn't do anything for himself —except drink. I washed his clothes and fixed his meals. I never brought my school friends around the house for fear that he would be drinking. Once I got my driver's license, I had to drive him to work and to the doctor. God, I feel like I never really had a father to take care of me. I was always taking care of him. That's my role in life—I end up taking care of people."

CAUSAL THEORY CONCLUSION: MOTHER

"She was alcoholic, too. I took care of her as well. She never asked what I needed, it was always what *she* wanted. I never knew what I needed. If I did, it wouldn't have done any good. I had to take care of both of my parents. I learned early that what I wanted didn't matter."

a. Construct a transference hypothesis that designates the most serious interpersonal problem:

_____

_____

_____

b. Identify the implicated transference domain: _____

Check your work with the criterion answers on p. 178.

Criterion Answers for Part II, Section C, Exercises

Transference Hypothesis 1

   a. *"If* I fail or make a mistake around Dr. Davis, *then* she will punish or reject me."

   b. Failure/mistakes.

Transference Hypothesis 2

   a. *"If* I get close to Dr. Hayes, *then* he will reject me or get mad at me for some reason—the relationship will not last."

   b. Intimacy/closeness.

Transference Hypothesis 3

   a. *"If* I make a mistake or don't do the right thing around Dr. Smith, *then* I'll have to hide it or she will punish or reject me."

   b. Failure/mistake.

Transference Hypothesis 4

   a. From father and mother: *"If* I get close to Dr. Emory, *then* I'll have to take care of him in some way."

   b. Intimacy/closeness.

     Note: A second transference hypothesis is indirectly suggested by the causal theory conclusions deduced from both the father and the mother: *"If* I need anything, *then* I'll not get it from Dr. Emory because I have to meet his needs" (Emotional need).

PART III
Interpersonal Discrimination Exercise

Once the transference hypotheses are formulated, the practitioner is ready to administer the Interpersonal Discrimination Exercise (IDE). This exercise can be administered whenever you move into a transference "hot spot" (review the text, pp. 91, 93–98). A good rule of thumb to follow is to administer the IDE task either *before* or *after* the SA work has been completed. Interrupting the SA with additional material always mitigates the behavioral consequence impact of the technique.

Several examples of transference "hot spots," when the IDE could be appropriately administered, are described below:

Transference domain	In-therapy events
1. Intimacy/closeness	Patient shares early sexual experiences with therapist; patient discloses affectionate feelings toward the therapist; patient and therapist work closely together at some task.
2. Emotional needs/problems	Patient is obviously frightened and doesn't know how to confront his/her spouse concerning the spouse's hurtful behavior; patient is grieved over the break-up of a longstanding love affair; patient loses job following illness.
3. Failure/mistakes	Patient forgets to bring in homework for the first time; patient is 15 minutes late for appointment; patient forgets the appointment and misses it; patient comes to session with a dark brown coffee stain across the front of his/her white shirt; patient fails when he/she attempts to carry out an agreed-upon homework assignment.
4. Negative affect felt/expressed	Patient impulsively says the therapist is frustrating him/her; patient gets mad at therapist in sudden outburst; patient tells therapist that he/she is wrong; patient looks angry after a statement by the therapist; patient becomes silent after disclosing an event in which significant shame has been communicated.

DIRECTIONS FOR ADMINISTERING THE IDE

1. Highlight the "hot spot" by describing what has just happened between the practitioner and the patient. For example: "You just expressed that you genuinely liked working

with me when we completed the SA you brought in today. Let's focus on what has just happened between us for a moment." (The *intimacy/closeness transference hypothesis* of being rejected if the patient gets close to Dr. Smith was previously formulated.)

2. Once the event is highlighted, the clinician then calls the name of the significant other(s) implicated in the causal theory conclusion(s) (i.e., mother, father, sibling, etc.) and inquires:

> "What would your mother have done had you said to her what you just said to me about liking to work with me?"

3. The patient is encouraged to describe in detail one or more memories when a similar event occurred with the mother. (Frequently, increased discomfort/distress will be observable in the patient.)

4. Once the mother's reactions (behavioral consequences) have been described, the clinician then asks the second question:

> "What was my reaction to you when you said this to me?"

The patient is encouraged to describe the therapist's reactions to her in as much detail as possible. If the patient appears unable to describe the clinician's behaviors, assistance is provided by the practitioner. It is important that both verbal/nonverbal behaviors are clearly pinpointed.

5. Then the *interpersonal discrimination question* is asked:

> "How do our reactions compare? Compare and contrast the similarities and the differences."

Time is allowed for the patient to compare and contrast the two behavioral consequences for the same behavior. (It is not unusual to see decreases in discomfort at this point, as it becomes clear that the clinician has not responded in a manner similar to the mother.)

6. A final discrimination question is asked:

> "What are the interpersonal implications for us, given the fact that I have not reacted to you in a hurtful, negative way when you got close to me?"

Again, the patient is given sufficient time to articulate the new implications that have just been presented to him/her.

When the IDE exercise is completed, the patient should be able to discriminate between the negative behavior of the significant other(s) and the positive behaviors of the clinician. Over the course of treatment, the message of IDE work becomes progressively clearer: *"With me, you have a new interpersonal reality on your hands. I will teach you to relate to me in novel and self-productive ways."*

Exercises

Following are six IDE exercises. For each:

1. Review the transference hypothesis for the patient.
2. Read the therapist-patient interaction and indicate if a transference "hot spot" is present.
3. *Check your work with the criterion answers on p. 185.*

IDE Exercise 1

TRANSFERENCE HYPOTHESIS

"*If* I make a mistake around Dr. Fowler, *then* he will reject/punish me for my foolish ways."

THERAPIST–PATIENT INTERACTION

THERAPIST: Why don't you tell me what happened last night with your girlfriend.

PATIENT: We went to a movie and had a good time together. I stayed over at her house last night, and it was wonderful. We both felt that we were closer last night than we have ever been before.

Is a transference "hot spot" indicated in the above conversation between the therapist and the patient?

Yes _____ No _____

Check your work with the criterion answers on p. 185.

IDE Exercise 2

TRANSFERENCE HYPOTHESIS

"*If* I need anything emotionally from Dr. Ryan, *then* she will not give it to me."

THERAPIST–PATIENT INTERACTION

PATIENT: I am scared to tell my editor what she has been doing to me.

THERAPIST: What do you mean?

PATIENT: She has been criticizing my work at every turn. Everything I do is wrong. It's getting so that I am afraid to turn in anything I write. When I turn in a piece of work, I am literally shaking when she takes it from me. You and I have worked on what I must say to her and how it's got to be said. I'm just scared to do it."

Is a transference "hot spot" indicated in the conversation between the therapist and the patient?

Yes _____   No _____

Check your work with the criterion answers on p. 185.

IDE Exercise 3

TRANSFERENCE HYPOTHESIS

"*If* I ever let Dr. Arrington know that I am angry with him, *then* he will kick me out of his office and not let me come back."

THERAPIST–PATIENT INTERACTION

THERAPIST: I need to reschedule our appointment for next week. I have to go to my daughter's soccer game next Thursday afternoon at 4 P.M. Can you come earlier in the day, or would it be more convenient if we got together on Friday morning?

PATIENT: (*looking very frustrated*) You just changed our meeting time the week before. I had to talk to my boss about getting off at a different time, and he didn't like it. I've never told him why I'm taking off—I'd rather not get into that with him, because I don't think he will understand. I thought that we had settled on this time as a regular appointment. (*long silence*) I will not be able to reschedule next week. (*Patient's voice sounding more irritated, but patient is trying to maintain composure.*) I need to work out a time when we can meet on a regular basis. Is this possible?

Is a transference "hot spot" indicated in the conversation between the therapist and the patient?

Yes _____   No _____

Check your work with the criterion answers on p. 185.

IDE Exercise 4

TRANSFERENCE HYPOTHESIS

"*If* I get close to Dr. Murray, *then* she will reject me."

THERAPIST–PATIENT INTERACTION

(*Patient is speaking*) "I've never worked things out with anyone before like you and I have done today. Every time I've gotten upset or in a mess in the past, I've left the room, broken off the relationship, or done something stupid to make things worse. Here you and I have taken a difficult situation that I mishandled badly. I lost my temper and really made an ass out of myself with my professor. Somehow, I've been able to stay in this seat and get through all my urges to leave. I've stayed and now I see a way to work out the mess I've got on my hands at the college. We have really done something together, really worked together, and that is very new for me. I feel really good about us right now."

Is a transference "hot spot" indicated in the conversation between the therapist and the patient?

Yes _____ No _____

Check your work with the criterion answers on p. 185.

IDE Exercise 5

TRANSFERENCE HYPOTHESIS

"*If* I make a mistake with Dr. Smothers, *then* she will punish me (like my parents did)."

THERAPIST–PATIENT INTERACTION

PATIENT: God, I left my Situational Analysis sheet on the dining-room table. I don't remember the situation I wrote out, and I can't think of a situation to work on here.

THERAPIST: We can figure something out. You seem very upset about having left the SA at home.

PATIENT: (*beginning to cry*) I've really messed up here. I'm so sorry. I guess you think I'm stupid for crying and all. I just can't help it. I've wanted to do everything right, and here I go, screwing up again.

Is a transference "hot spot" indicated in the conversation between the therapist and the patient?

Yes _____ No _____

Check your work with the criterion answers on p. 185.

IDE Exercise 6

TRANSFERENCE HYPOTHESIS

"*If* I need anything emotionally from Dr. Cole, *then* she will withdraw from me and I will not get it."

THERAPIST–PATIENT INTERACTION

THERAPIST: Tell me how your week has gone.

PATIENT: I finally asserted myself to my boyfriend. He was beginning to talk to me in that rude tone of voice the other night while we were out. I didn't hold back. I told him that I didn't like the sound of his voice, that it was rude and ugly. I also said to him that if he continued speaking to me in that tone of voice that I wanted him to take me home. God, did he stop. He even apologized! I can't believe I did this. It's the first time I stood up for myself.

Is a transference "hot spot" indicated in the conversation between the therapist and the patient?

Yes _____   No _____

Check your work with the criterion answers on the facing page.

Criterion Answers for Part III Exercises

IDE Exercise 1

No. There is no mistake situation indicated in the conversation and the transference hypothesis "hot spot" is not implicated.

IDE Exercise 2

Yes. The patient is talking about a fear-engendering situation that she must confront with her editor. The transference hypothesis states that whenever she needs emotional support or some other emotional assistance from Dr. Ryan, she will not receive what she needs. The practitioner must provide the emotional support, and the stage will then be set for the administration of the IDE. The transference hypothesis "hot spot" of needing emotional support is clearly implicated.

IDE Exercise 3

Yes. The patient is obviously frustrated and angry with Dr. Arrington. The change of appointment times is translating into problems between the patient and his boss, which is stressful and embarrassing. The patient is trying to maintain emotional control, but the frustration and anger is nonverbally leaking through in his conversation with Dr. Arrington. After the appointment issue has been settled, Dr. Arrington is in an optimal position to conduct an IDE with the patient, now that the transference hypothesis "hot spot" is implicated.

IDE Exercise 4

Yes. The patient and Dr. Murray have accomplished a "first" in the life of this patient. It has ended with a positive outcome and the patient makes a comment to Dr. Murray that is endearing (i.e., "I feel really good about us right now"). The stage is set for IDE administration because the intimacy/closeness transference hypothesis is implicated.

IDE Exercise 5

Yes. Dr. Smothers has a situation of "failure" on her hands that implicates the transference hypothesis. The patient has obviously tried to do things "right" in therapy, and this event signals that her well-laid plans, because of her mistake, have not worked out. The IDE will demonstrate to the patient that the parents' punishment for her failings do not occur with this therapist. Such occasions often turn out to be corrective emotional experiences for patients.

IDE Exercise 6

No. The transference hypothesis denotes emotional need. The situation between Dr. Cole and the patient involves something quite different. The patient reports a successful assertive event that she produced with her boyfriend. The transference hypothesis is not implicated, and the IDE will have to be used later when an exchange involving emotional need occurs.

References

American Psychiatric Association. (1994). *Diagnostic and Statistical Manual of Mental Disorders (4th ed.).* Washington, DC: Author.

Beck, A. T., Rush, A. J., Shaw, B. F., & Emery, G. (1979). *Cognitive Therapy of Depression.* New York: Guilford Press.

Cowan, P. A. (1978). *Piaget with Feeling: Cognitive, Social, and Emotional Dimensions.* New York: Holt, Rinehart & Winston.

Gordon, D. E. (1988). Formal operations and interpersonal and affective disturbances in adolescents. In E. D. Nannis & P. A. Cowan (Eds.), *Developmental Psychopathology and Its Treatment* (pp. 51–73). San Francisco: Jossey-Bass.

Horwitz, J. A. (2001). *Early-onset versus late-onset chronic depressive disorders: Comparison of retrospective reports of coping with adversity in the childhood home environment.* Unpublished master's thesis, Department of Psychology, Virginia Commonwealth University, Richmond.

Inhelder, B., & Piaget, J. (1958). *The Growth of Logical Thinking from Childhood to Adolescence.* New York: Basic Books. (Original work published 1955)

Keller, M. B. (1988). Diagnostic issues and clinical course of unipolar illness. In A. J. Frances & R. E. Hales (Eds.), *Review of Psychiatry* (Vol. 7, pp. 188–212). Washington, DC: American Psychiatric Press.

Keller, M. B. (1990). Diagnostic and course-of-illness variables pertinent to refractory depression. In A. Tasman, S. M. Goldfinger, & C. A. Kaufman (Eds.), *Review of Psychiatry* (Vol. 9, pp. 10–32). Washington, DC: American Psychiatric Press.

Keller, M. B., & Hanks, D. L. (1994). The natural history and heterogeneity of depressive disorders. *Journal of Clinical Psychiatry, 56,* 22–29.

Keller, M. B., Klein, D. N., Hirschfeld, R. M. A., Kocsis, J. H., McCullough, J. P., Miller, I., First, M. B., Holzer, C. P., III, Keitner, G. I., Marin, D. B., & Shea, T. (1995). Results of the *DSM-IV* mood disorders field trial. *American Journal of Psychiatry, 152,* 843–849.

Keller, M. B., Lavori, P. W., Rice, J., Coryell, W., & Hirschfeld, R. M. A. (1986). The persistent risk of chronicity in recurrent episodes of nonbipolar major depressive disorder: A prospective follow-up. *American Journal of Psychiatry, 143,* 24–28.

Keller, M. B., McCullough, J. P., Klein, D. N., Arnow, B., Dunner, D. L., Gelenberg, A. J., Markowitz, J. C., Nemeroff, C. B., Russell, J. M., Thase, M. E., Trivedi, M. H., & Zajecka, J. (2000). A comparison of nefazodone, the Cognitive Behavioral Analysis System of Psychotherapy, and their combination for the treatment of chronic depression. *New England Journal of Medicine, 342,* 1462–1470.

Keller, M. B., & Shapiro, R. W. (1982). Double depression: Superimposition of acute depressive episodes on chronic depressive disorders. *American Journal of Psychiatry, 139*, 438–442.

Keller, M. B., & Shapiro, R. W. (1984). Double depression, major depression, and dysthymia: Distinct entities or different phases of a single disorder? *Psychopathology Bulletin, 20*, 399–402.

Kiesler, D. J. (1983). The 1982 Interpersonal Circle: A taxonomy for complementarity in human transactions. *Psychological Review, 90*, 185–214.

Kiesler, D. J. (1987). *Research Manual for the Impact Message Inventory*. Palo Alto, CA: Consulting Psychologist Press.

Kiesler, D. J. (1996). *Contemporary Interpersonal Theory and Research: Personality, Psychopathology, and Psychotherapy*. New York: Wiley.

Kiesler, D. J., & Schmidt, J. A. (1993). *The Impact Message Inventory: Form IIA Octant Scale Version*. Redwood City, CA: Mind Garden.

McCullough, J. P. (1984). Cognitive-behavioral analysis system of psychotherapy: An interactional treatment approach for dysthymia disorder. *Psychiatry, 47*, 234–250.

McCullough, J. P. (2000). *Treatment for Chronic Depression: Cognitive Behavioral Analysis System of Psychotherapy*. New York: Guilford Press.

McCullough, J. P., Kornstein, S. G., McCullough, J. P., Belyea- Caldwell, S., Kaye, A. L., Roberts, W. C., Plybon, J. K., & Kruus, L. K. (1996). Differential diagnosis of chronic depressive disorders. *The Psychiatric Clinics of North America, 19*, 55–71.

McCullough, J. P., McCune, K. J., Kaye, A. L., Braith, J. A., Friend, R., Roberts, W. C., Belyea-Caldwell, S., Norris, S. L. W., & Hampton, C. (1994). One-year prospective replication study of an untreated sample of community dysthymia subjects. *Journal of Nervous and Mental Disease, 182*, 396–401.

Nannis, E. D. (1988). Cognitive-developmental differences in emotional understanding. In E. D. Nannis & P. A. Cowan (Eds.), *Developmental Psychopathology and Its Treatment* (pp. 31–49). San Francisco: Jossey-Bass.

Piaget, J. (1926). *The Language and Thought of the Child*. New York: Harcourt, Brace. (Original work published 1923)

Piaget, J. (1981). *Intelligence and Affectivity: Their Relationship during Child Development*. Palo Alto, CA: Annual Reviews. (Original work published 1954)

Skinner, B. F. (1956). A case history in scientific method. *American Psychologist, 11*, 221–233.